NINE MONTHS AND COUNTING

NINE MONTHS

& COUNTING

BIBLE PROMISES AND BRIGHT IDEAS
FOR PREGNANCY AND AFTER

by ALICE CHAPIN

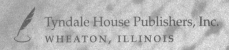
Tyndale House Publishers, Inc.
WHEATON, ILLINOIS

Visit Tyndale's exciting Web site at www.tyndale.com

Edited by Chimena Kabasenche

Designed by Melinda Schumacher

Scripture quotations marked KJV are taken from the *Holy Bible,* King James Version.

Scripture quotations marked NIV are taken from the *Holy Bible,* New International Version®. NIV®. Copyright © 1973, 1978, 1984 by International Bible Society. Used by permission of Zondervan Publishing House. All rights reserved.

Scripture quotations marked NLT are taken from the *Holy Bible,* New Living Translation, copyright © 1996. Used by permission of Tyndale House Publishers, Inc., Wheaton, Illinois 60189. All rights reserved.

Scripture quotations marked NRSV are taken from the New Revised Standard Version of the Bible, copyrighted, 1989 by the Division of Christian Education of the National Council of the Churches of Christ in the United States of America, and are used by permission. All rights reserved.

The One Year Book of Hymns, copyright © 1995 by Robert K. Brown and Mark R. Norton. All rights reserved. Used by permission. *The One Year* is a registered trademark of Tyndale House Publishers, Inc.

Carol Van Klompenburg's poems, "Did I conceive a child?" and "Birth/One final push . . ." are from *Loving Your Preborn Baby,* Carol Van Klompenburg, copyright, Harold Shaw Publishers, Wheaton, Illinois. All rights reserved. Used by permission.

The Billy Graham quote is from *Angels,* Billy Graham, copyright, Word Publishing, Nashville, Tennessee. All rights reserved. Used by permission.

The Maja Bernath quote is from *Parents' Book for Your Baby's First Year,* Maja Bernath, copyright © 1983, Ballantine Books, New York, New York. All rights reserved. Used by permission.

Life Application Bible, copyright © 1988, 1989, 1990, 1991 by Tyndale House Publishers, Inc., Wheaton, IL 60189. All rights reserved. Used by permission. *Life Application* is a registed trademark of Tyndale House Publishers, Inc.

TouchPoint Bible, copyright © 1996 by Tyndale House Publishers, Inc., Wheaton, IL 60189. All rights reserved. Used by permission. *TouchPoint* is a registered trademark of Tyndale House Publishers, Inc.

Library of Congress Cataloging-in-Publication Data

Chapin, Alice Zillman.
  Nine months and counting : Bible promises and bright ideas for pregnancy and after / by Alice Chapin.
    p.   cm.
  ISBN 0-8423-7363-2 (sc : alk. paper)
  1. Pregnant women—Religious life.   2. Pregnancy—Religious aspects—Christianity.   I. Title.
BV4529.18.C43   1999
248.8'431—dc21   99-26601

Printed in the United States of America

06 05 04 03 02
8   7   6   5   4   3   2

*"Babies are such a nice way
to start people."*

DON HEROLD

TABLE OF CONTENTS

FOREWORD

❦

So, you're having a baby!

You are about to participate in an incredible event, possibly the most profound experience that can happen to a woman. One person becomes two—something too wonderful for words!

Birthing a child is surely a divine process. Who can explain how the human body achieves such a task? The life-forming process of birth is certainly planned elsewhere, but it occurs inside the womb. After conception, the woman's body takes over the tremendously complicated pregnancy procedure without direction from her. God's hand is the key to this pattern. Who else but God could direct all of a woman's strength and resources to order millions of new cells into existence from nowhere and to mobilize them in about sixty-four hundred hours (thirty-eight weeks)? Who else but God could produce a wonderfully functioning new little person with hands, feet, eyes, ears, a brain, and a nervous system? The mother's body is the container God uses to hold, nurture, and shape this brand-new human being. The sacred dimensions are so obvious, so numerous, so mysterious that childbirth must be called a holy act.

That's why I have included so many Bible passages and devotional thoughts in this book. But that's not all! I have also incorporated dozens of bright ideas and practical suggestions—all from seasoned moms who have learned to cope creatively on the journey into motherhood. Also included are helpful things for you to do and to know when preparing for Baby. And there is also room for Mom to write down her thoughts and experiences both while carrying her child and after the child is born.

I am praying that your pregnancy will be filled with joyful anticipation and good health and that your newborn child will be a delight to you. "May the Lord richly bless both you and your children" (Psalm 115:14, NLT).

Happy mothering!

With love,

Alice Chapin

Alice Chapin
Newnan, Georgia

Be fruitful, and multiply.

GENESIS 1:28, KJV

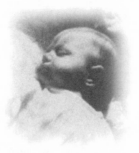

MOM'S PROFILE

In years to come, it will be very interesting to take a look at what you were like back then while carrying your baby. Changes up ahead are bound to make you a very different person, maybe even a much better person. Old hobbies, interests, and habits are often left behind as new ones appear. Here is your chance, Mom, to record your life as it is right now. You'll be glad you did. And won't your grandchildren love having a word portrait painted by Grandma herself?

My birthdate: _____

Today's date: _____

My height: _____

Eye color: _____

Hair color: _____

Place of birth: _____

The most important values in my life right now are: _____

_____

My four highest priorities in order of their importance are: _____

_____

_____

_____

The people most responsible for who I am today are: _____

_____

Because: _____

Two things that make me happy are: _____

Things that make me angry are: _____

The biggest and best dream I have for myself is: _____

The biggest and best dream I have for my baby is: _____

If I could speak to my baby now, I would say: _____

My favorite foods are: _____

My favorite kinds of music are: _____

Musical instruments I can play: _____

How well? _____

Favorite instrument? musician? singer? music group? _____

My favorite colors are: _____

My favorite author is: _____

Favorite book? poem? movie? television program? magazine?

_____

_____

A favorite quote: _____

_____

Who said or wrote it? _____

The loveliest word I can think of is: _____

A word that irks me is: _____

Some things that make me laugh are: _____

_____

Three of my favorite possessions are: _____

Because: _____

_____

The most satisfying thing in my life right now is: _____

_____

The main worry in my life right now is: _____

_____

My favorite hobbies or things to do are: _____

_____

My least favorite thing to do is: _____

_____

Clubs or organizations I belong to are: _____

_____

My pet peeve is: _____

My favorite flower is: _____

Favorite leaf? tree? land feature? animal? _____

_____

The things I like best about my family are: _____

_____

Some things my family disagrees on are: _____

_____

I have ___ have not ___ spent a lot of time around children before becoming pregnant.

Right now, my favorite age of a child seems to be: _____

_____

How do I feel about wearing the maternity clothes I have bought or borrowed: Privileged or run-of-the-mill? beautiful or plain? classy or dowdy? excited and filled with joy or afraid and nervous? glad the world now knows about Baby—or wishing it were still a secret?

_____

_____

_____

Something that has made me feel sad or disappointed lately is:

_____

How I handled it: _____

_____

Something that has made me feel anxious lately is: _____

_____

Some fears I used to have that have disappeared are: _____

_____

Why these went away: _____

_____

Three of my best qualities are: _____

_____

The achievements I am most proud of in my life are: _____

_____

A mistake I made in my life has been: _____

_____

What I have done about it: _____

_____

If I could go back and change something in my life, I would:

_____

_____

One of the most awful days in my life was: _____

_____

How I survived: _____

_____

A time when something humorous or ironic happened was:

_____

_____

_____

_____

Changes I need to make in my life because I am about to become
somebody's mother are: _____

The kind of woman I am working on becoming is: _____

_____

A woman I admire very much is: _____

Because: _____

A man I admire very much is: _____

Because: _____

A mother I especially admire is:_____

Because: _____

A father I especially admire is: _____

Because: _____

I think I will make a good mother because: _____

_____

If I could change places with someone today, I would choose:

_____

Because: _____

My best friend's name is:_____

How we know each other: _____

How I feel about things in today's world (in a nutshell):

Human sexuality: _____

Abortion: _____

Media and entertainment: _____

Our government: _____

Marriage and divorce:_____

Public schools: _____

Poverty: _____

Technology: _____

Church: _____

Environment: _____

Sometimes I wish: _____

_____

If I could change the world for my baby, I would: _____

_____

_____

An important goal I have for my family's life together in the years ahead is: _____

_____

Today, I am especially thankful for: _____

_____

The best thing that happened to me this week is: _____

_____

This year: _____

In my lifetime: _____

Something about me that few people know (dreams, desires, or accomplishments) is: _____

_____

Some remembrances about my mother are: _____

_____

Some remembrances about my father are: _____

_____

Some remembrances about my grandparents are: _____

_____

Some remembrances about my extended family (cousins, aunts,
uncles, nieces, nephews, others) are: _____

_____

_____

Some remembrances about my siblings are: _____

_____

_____

The five people I love most are: _____

_____

Five people who love me are: _____

_____

I am being good to myself these days by: _____

_____

I need to forgive myself for: _____

_____

The church I attend is: _____

Describe: _____

Member? _____

Baptized? when? by whom? _____

_____

A few sentences describing how I came to believe in Jesus Christ:

_____

_____

_____

Someone who has helped me and encouraged me in the Christian life is: _____

How did they help and encourage me? _____

_____

My favorite Scriptures are: _____

_____

Because: _____

_____

When I feel God is far away, I: _____

_____

When I feel close to God, I: _____

_____

Things I most want my baby to know about God are (include Scripture references): _____

_____

One way I have been spiritually challenged or convicted lately is:

_____

_____

Some times when I have experienced God's protection or provision for me are: _____

The prayer I most often pray is: _____

I believe God's purpose in creating me and other people on earth is:

_____

_____

Why I believe this: _____

Today, I need special prayer for: _____

_____

I do __ do not __ fear death because: _____

_____

I believe heaven belongs to those who: _____

_____

I believe in these truths: _____

_____

_____

Struggles I have had with faith and God are: _____

_____

_____

I know God understands me because: _____

_____

My favorite popular personality is: _____

My favorite religious personality is: _____

Someone who showed love for me this week is: _____

How was love shown? _____

How I showed love to someone else this week: _____

_____

Here is a prayer for my baby: _____

_____

_____

MAKING

THE

ADJUSTMENT

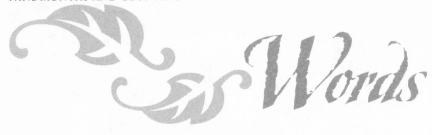

Therefore shall a man leave his father and his mother, and shall cleave unto his wife: and they shall be one flesh. And they were both naked, the man and his wife, and were not ashamed.

GENESIS 2:24-25, KJV

God said, "Let us make people. . . ." Male and female he created them. God blessed them and told them, "Multiply and fill the earth."

GENESIS 1:26-28, NLT

We are God's masterpiece. He has created us anew in Christ Jesus.

EPHESIANS 2:10, NLT

As you do not know the path of the wind, or how the body is formed in a mother's womb, so you cannot understand the work of God, the Maker of all things.

ECCLESIASTES 11:5, NIV

to Live By

There is a time for everything, a season for every activity under heaven. A time to be born and a time to die. A time to plant and a time to harvest. A time to cry and a time to laugh.

ECCLESIASTES 3:1-2, 4, NLT

God places the lonely in families.

PSALM 68:6, NLT

The Lord gave me a message. He said, "I knew you before I formed you in your mother's womb."

JEREMIAH 1:4-5, NLT

I will meditate on your wonderful miracles.

PSALM 119:27, NLT

Mary reacts prayerfully and with willingness as the Lord's servant when told of her pregnancy:

Don't be frightened, Mary," the angel told her, "for God has decided to bless you! You will become pregnant and have a son, and you are to name him Jesus. He will be very great and will be called the Son of the Most High. . . ."

Mary asked the angel, "But how can I have a baby? I am a virgin."

The angel replied, "The Holy Spirit will come upon you, and the power of the Most High will overshadow you. So the baby born to you will be holy, and he will be called the Son of God. . . ."

Mary responded, "I am the Lord's servant, and I am willing to accept whatever he wants. May everything you have said come true."

[Later:] Because Joseph was a descendent of King David, he had to go to Bethlehem in Judea, David's ancient home [for the census]. . . . He took with him Mary, his fiancée, who was obviously pregnant. . . . And while they were there . . . she gave birth to her first child, a son. She wrapped him snugly in strips of cloth and laid him in a manger, because there was no room for them in the village inn.

LUKE 1:30-38; 2:4-7, NLT

The Magnificat: Mary's Song of Praise
"Oh, how I praise the Lord.
  How I rejoice in God my Savior!
For he took notice of his lowly servant girl,
   and now generation after generation
   will call me blessed.
For he, the Mighty One, is holy,
   and he has done great things for me.
His mercy goes on from generation to generation,
   to all who fear him.
His mighty arm does tremendous things!
   How he scatters the proud and haughty ones!
He has taken princes from their thrones
   and exalted the lowly."

LUKE 1:46-52, NLT

Our days on earth are like grass; like wildflowers, we bloom and die. The wind blows, and we are gone— as though we had never been here. But the love of the Lord remains forever with those who fear him. His salvation extends to the children's children of those who are faithful to his covenant, of those who obey his commandments!

PSALM 103:15-18, NLT

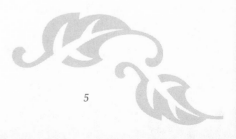

"Worth Repeating"

"If my first child had known that she was absolutely dependent upon a mother who felt completely helpless and inadequate, she may not have slept so soundly and sweetly in her bassinet those first few weeks."

"It is incredible when we think how little our parents knew about child psychology and how wonderful we turned out to be!"

"Conceiving and bringing forth a new life is a divine experience, a powerful encounter with the God of the universe. Growing a human being inside is a holy time."

"Not only am I giving birth to a baby, I am also giving birth to a mother."

"God is the maker of all things. He is the supervisor of this intricate project called pregnancy. I am his partner in growing this brand-new life inside. It is almost as if he has borrowed my body for nine months to form this child. Whether I am religious or not, discern him or not, God is there."

"Babies may be deductible, but they are still taxing."

"Wanted: Baby carrier, car seat, playpen, high chair—and cot. Also: two single beds (for temporary use only)."

"When God wants an important thing done in this world or a wrong righted, he doesn't release thunderbolts or stir up earthquakes. He simply has a tiny baby born, perhaps in a very humble home, perhaps of a very humble mother. And he puts it in the baby's mind, and then God waits. The great events of this world are babies."

EDWARD MCDONALD

"Children are gifts, if we accept them."

KATHLEEN TIERNEY CRILLY

"A recent story tells about a baby who was giggling and laughing minutes after he was born. The obstetrician noticed that the newborn had unusual muscle control, his tiny left fist being tightly clenched. When the doctor pried it open, he found a contraceptive pill."

EVAN ESAR

"Do not pray for easy lives. Pray to be strong men [and women]. Do not pray for tasks equal to your powers but for powers equal to your tasks. Then the doing of your work will be no miracle, but you shall be a miracle. Every day you shall wonder at yourself, at the richness of your life which has come to you by the grace of God."

PHILLIPS BROOKS

"Whenever I hear people discussing birth control, I always remember that I was the fifth."

CLARENCE DARROW

"When you have a baby, you set off an explosion in your marriage, and when the dust settles, your marriage is different from what it was. Not better, necessarily; not worse, necessarily, but different."

NORA EPHRON

"It is not that I half knew my mother. I knew half of her: the lower half—her lap, legs, feet, her hands and wrists as she bent forward."

FLANN O'BRIEN

"A young mother with a baby in her arms is ever a means of drawing human thoughts toward that Mother and that Babe who stand forever as our conception of the meeting point of earth and heaven."

UNKNOWN

"It's like you grow another heart, like someone kicks
down a door that was sealed shut, and then the whole
world—sunshine, flowers—falls through."

Rosie O'Donnell

"Did I conceive a child?
or, child,
by forming
did you conceive a mother?"

Carol Van Klompenburg, *Loving Your Preborn Baby*

"Drop thy still dews of quietness,
Till all our strivings cease;
Take from our souls the strain and stress,
And let our ordered lives confess
The beauty of thy peace."

John Greenleaf Whittier

THINGS TO KNOW

The act of conceiving a baby may seem simple to the two people involved, but inside, conception is the beginning of an arduous journey. Upon their release, up to two hundred million sperm beat their tails in a desperate race through the woman's uterus toward her fallopian tubes, where a single fertile egg lies waiting. Only a few hundred will make it to the fallopian tubes, and about one-tenth of those will crowd in a wiggling halo around their quarry, eagerly seeking admission. One penetrates, and instantly all other suitors are excluded by the egg's special membrane.

IRENA CHALMERS

The one sperm that achieves its destiny has won against gigantic odds, several hundred million to one. The baby it engenders has a far greater mathematical chance of becoming president than the sperm had of fathering a baby.

ALAN GUTTMACHER, M.D.

Galen, a second-century Greek physician, came up with the idea that all women carry within them well-formed microscopic fetuses in a sac. He believed that semen caused one or two of these mini-mini-babies to break out of their embryonic capsule and grow inside the mother for nine months until ready for birth.

Many researchers say that babies recognize their own mother's voice after birth. One mother, who sang the old hymn "Constantly Abiding" over and over to her unborn son, says that as a child he often whistled the tune. It remains his favorite hymn, even though he is now grown.

Sit by yourself today and

imagine God at work

forming the new life inside you, cell by cell:

baby's head, eyes, ears, inner parts, skin, legs, feet.

Surely, if we could watch it happening

with our eyes, we would fall on our knees

at our heavenly Father's feet!

I became more sensitive to others, more aware of their needs, when I had a baby to look after. Before, I now admit, I was a selfish person, always trying to meet my own needs and desires. After Baby, my heart shifted. I became milder in nature, more patient, more willing to give up what I wanted. I call that learning to love. Isn't that what Jesus himself said was the most important thing in the world—to love?

If God cares enough about an unborn child to personally schedule his or her days, shouldn't we also have a sense of holy care for unborn children? God's continued presence demonstrates a strong and holy love for this developing person. Can we do less?

THE *TouchPoint Bible* ON PSALM 139

You, O Lord, will rule forever. Your fame will endure to every generation. . . . Let this be recorded for future generations, so that a nation yet to be created will praise the Lord. . . . They will fade away. But you are always the same; your years never end. The children of your people will live in security. Their children's children will thrive in your presence.

PSALM 102:12, 18, 26-28, NLT

Time with God

God and I together are growing a human, with blood and muscle and bone and brain—a sacred being—someone who bears his own image and who will breathe and cry and eat and have feelings in due time. The person who comes forth will likely join God in growing yet another human being who will beget yet another and another. Life goes on. And I am part of this intriguing and never-ending chain of people and events.

There probably isn't anything harder to do than wait, whether we are expecting something good, something bad, or an unknown.

One way we often cope with a long wait is to begin helping God get his plan into action. Sarah tried this approach. She was too old to expect to have a child of her own, so she thought God must have something else in mind. From Sarah's limited point of view, this could only be to give Abraham a son through another woman—a common practice in her day. The plan seemed harmless enough. Abraham would sleep with Sarah's servant, who would then give birth to a child. Sarah would take the child as her own. The plan worked beautifully—at first. But as you read about the events that followed, you will be struck by how often Sarah must have regretted the day she decided to push God's timetable ahead.

What parts of your life seem to be on hold right now? Do you understand that this may be part of God's plan for you? The Bible has more than enough clear direction to keep us busy while we're waiting for some particular part of life to move ahead.

Life Application Bible, "SARAH" SKETCH IN GENESIS 18

During pregnancy, my baby and I are under the heavenly Father's care. One of the Bible names given him is El Shaddai which means Almighty God, Strengthener, Satisfier, Makes Fruitful (Genesis 17: 1). Can I doubt a God like this? He says, "I am the Lord; that is my name!" (Isaiah 42:8, NLT).

Prayer & Meditation

Speak, Lord, in the stillness,

While I wait on Thee;

Hushed my heart to listen

In expectancy.

Speak, O blessed Master,

In this quiet hour,

Let me see Thy face, Lord,

Feel Thy touch of power.

The One Year Book of Hymns, SEPTEMBER 5

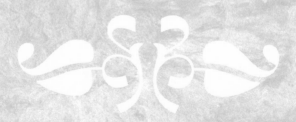

Envision God looking down with love upon you and your baby inside. Ask God to bestow health, wonderful abilities and talents, and a pleasant temperament on your baby. You can begin to pray today for Baby to love God, for good friends and teachers, and even for a perfect mate for a lifetime.

Thank the Lord today for the privilege of being a mother even though it involves being a servant to your child.

Think of other women you know who are now pregnant. Offer a prayer for them.

Pray for an opportunity to give some encouragement or comfort to someone else today. In your prayer be specific about someone you would like to help.

Things to Do
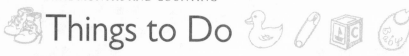

First Trimester,
Months One to Three

1. Talk to friends about the best healthcare provider, then select.
2. Make a first visit to the healthcare provider by the end of the third month.
3. Stop smoking, drinking alcohol, or taking any drugs that might be harmful to your baby. Ask your doctor if in doubt.
4. Ask about a proper eating program to ensure good health for Mother and Baby. Eat right for proper nutrition.
5. Check out prenatal and other pregnancy-related classes in the community, such as Lamaze or sibling orientation classes, etc.
6. Make a dental appointment.
7. Make a list of emergency phone numbers (doctor or midwife, hospital, ambulance, Dad's or a friend's workplace number, etc.).
8. Check stores and catalogs for maternity styles.

Second Trimester,
Months Four to Six

1. Sign up for childbirth education classes.
2. Buy (or borrow) and read books on pregnancy, labor and delivery, and care of newborns. Make decisions on things like breastfeeding, childbirth methods, circumcision, whom you want with you during delivery, whether you want your baby with you immediately after birth, and other important issues.
3. Begin shopping for Baby (see list on page 176).
4. Do any sewing you plan for yourself or for Baby's room.
5. Find out which symptoms to watch out for that might indicate a need for emergency or specialized care.
6. Shop for maternity clothes (see hints on page 108).

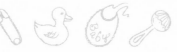   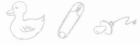

Third Trimester,
Months Seven to Nine

1. Select birth announcements. Envelopes can be addressed ahead of time.
2. Make a list of needed baby items in case people ask.
3. Make a list of people to phone after Baby comes.
4. Read books on care of newborns. Learn about health checks and procedures done on babies right after birth.
5. Pack a hospital bag.
6. Arrange for a diaper service if needed.
7. Make arrangements for a housekeeper or sitter for children or pets. Compile a list of responsibilities and other things helpers should know.
8. Finish arranging Baby's room.
9. Finish shopping for Baby.
10. Select a pediatrician. You will need one after birth. Ask friends for recommendations.
11. Prepare and freeze meals and treats for later.

Begin moving the older child from the crib to a bed several weeks before Baby arrives home. The sibling will probably consider it a privilege to use a grown-up bed instead of feeling pushed out of his old bed.

Present the youngster with her very own easy-to-use camera a few weeks ahead of Baby's arrival. Showing her how to load it and take pictures of the newborn will heighten the excitement.

Just for fun, plan a baby food taste-test game with older kids. Cover the labels of about a dozen jars of various kinds of baby food with masking or electrical tape. Number the jars and keep track of what is inside each. Let everyone write down a guess about the contents. The person who most often guesses correctly wins a gift certificate to Wendy's or McDonald's. Use plain, one-ingredient baby foods, not mixed foods like soups.

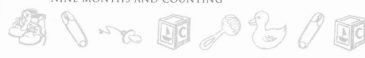

(To Mom: If you think this is easy, guess again. Food for babies often does not resemble adult food in either taste or color.)

Cut a silhouette outline of your child's head from black construction paper, then mount it on cardboard to be hung in Baby's room. To trace the outline, set the child in front of a sheet of white paper taped to the wall. Direct a bright light so that a shadow of your child's profile appears on the paper, and carefully mark along the edges of the shadow. Loosely tape the tracing to the black construction paper. Cut out your child's silhouette and mount it on the cardboard.

For a proud family pregnancy, make designer T-shirts announcing, *We're Having a Baby at Our House*, for Dad, Mom, and all the kids. Or stitch a message on everybody's socks. Run bright red ribbon along the top edges to attract attention. Maybe you can all wear your shirts and socks at a family picnic in the park so your group will stand out from everybody else's.

Let older children help you start a scrapbook to record a few important pregnancy events as they occur—things like how you told them and Baby's father you are pregnant, how siblings and grandparents reacted, and what family members have said. Write down how you chose a name, when you first felt Baby move, how you feel during this pregnancy, thoughts all of you have about Baby-to-be, important family events, and prayers for Baby and the other children. Add notes about what makes your family unique and the things each of you especially likes about your household. Later, record a few sentences about the birthing. This will make interesting reading in a few years.

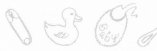

Kids' curiosity will peak when they see you putting up a bulletin board. Gather baby photographs of older siblings and of yourself and Dad. Tell the children it is part of a mystery project that Dad or someone else will be doing with them while you are in the hospital. (They will decorate and post family photographs while you are away.) Everyone will have fun raving over cute curly- or baldheaded baby pictures, especially Mom's and Dad's. When your newborn arrives home to become part of the family, the children can add their first photos and congratulation cards and letters to the bulletin board.

LIVING

IN

ANTICIPATION

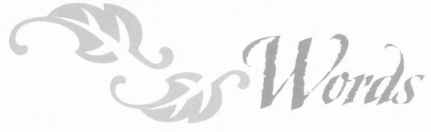

Words

Manoah and his wife ask guidance about Samson:

A man named Manoah . . . lived in the town of Zorah. His wife was unable to become pregnant, and they had no children. The angel of the Lord appeared to Manoah's wife and said, ". . .You must not drink wine or any other alcoholic drink or eat any forbidden food. You will become pregnant and give birth to a son, and his hair must never be cut. For he will be dedicated to God as a Nazirite from birth. He will rescue Israel from the Philistines."

Then Manoah prayed to the Lord. He said, "Lord, please let the man of God come back to us again and give us more instructions about this son who is to be born." God answered his prayer, and the angel of God appeared once again to his wife. . . . So Manoah asked him, "When your words come true, what kind of rules should govern the boy's life and work?" The angel of the Lord replied, "Be sure your wife follows the instructions I gave her. She must not eat grapes or raisins, drink wine or any other alcoholic drink, or eat any forbidden food. . . ."

When her son was born, they named him Samson. And the Lord blessed him as he grew up. And in Mahaneh-dan . . . the Spirit of the Lord began to take hold of him.

JUDGES 13:2-25, NLT, SELECTED VERSES

to Live By

Mary hurried to the hill country of Judea, to the town where Zechariah lived. She entered the house and greeted Elizabeth. At the sound of Mary's greeting, Elizabeth's child leaped within her.

LUKE 1:39-41, NLT

Hannah prays and God gives her Samuel:

[Hannah] was in bitterness of soul, and prayed unto the Lord, and wept sore. And she vowed a vow, and said, "O Lord of hosts, if thou wilt indeed look on the affliction of thine handmaid, and remember me, and not forget thine handmaid, but wilt give unto thine handmaid a man child, then I will give him unto the Lord all the days of his life. . . ." It came to pass, when the time was come about after Hannah had conceived, that she bare a son and called his name Samuel, saying, "Because I have asked him of the Lord. . . . For this child I prayed; and the Lord hath given me my petition. . . . Therefore . . . as long as he liveth he shall be lent to the Lord."

1 SAMUEL 1:10-11, 20, 27-28, KJV

25

[A Jewish priest] Zechariah and [his wife] Elizabeth were righteous in God's eyes. . . . They had no children because Elizabeth was barren, and now they were both very old.

One day Zechariah was serving God in the Temple. . . . As was the custom of the priests, he was chosen by lot to enter the sanctuary and burn incense in the Lord's presence. While the incense was being burned, a great crowd stood outside, praying. . . . An angel of the Lord appeared. . . . Zechariah was overwhelmed with fear. But the angel said, "Don't be afraid, Zechariah! For God has heard your prayer, and your wife, Elizabeth, will bear you a son! And you are to name him John. You will have great joy and gladness. . . . He will change disobedient minds to accept godly wisdom."

Soon afterward his wife, Elizabeth, became pregnant and went into seclusion for five months. "How kind the Lord is!" she exclaimed. "He has taken away my disgrace of having no children!"

LUKE 1:6-14, 17, 24, NLT

I created you and have cared for you since before you were born. I will be your God throughout your lifetime . . . . I made you, and I will care for you. I will carry you along.

ISAIAH 46:3-4, NLT

Whatever is good and perfect [babies too] comes to us from God above, who created all heaven's lights. . . .

JAMES 1:17, NLT

You both precede and follow me. You place your hand of
blessing on my head. Such knowledge is too wonderful for
me, too great for me to know!

PSALM 139:5-6, NLT

You made all the delicate, inner parts of my body and
knit me together in my mother's womb. You saw me
before I was born. Every day of my life was recorded in
your book. Every moment was laid out.

PSALM 139:13, 16, NLT

Our soul waiteth for the Lord; he is our help and our shield.

PSALM 33:20, KJV

I waited patiently for the Lord; he inclined to me and
heard my cry. He put a new song in my mouth, a song of
praise. . . . Happy are those who make the Lord their trust.

PSALM 40:1, 3-4, NRSV

Be still, and know that I am God; I will be exalted among
the nations, I will be exalted in the earth.

PSALM 46:10, NIV

In quietness and confidence is your strength.

ISAIAH 30:15, NLT

[God] has made everything beautiful in its time.

ECCLESIASTES 3:11, NIV

"Worth Repeating"

"How luxurious, pregnancy! A perfect universe mine to offer."

SUSAN EISENBERG

"How wise of God every twenty years to give us a new generation of children in the Church."

MARTIN LUTHER

"Mothering is never, never polished nor orderly nor placid nor smooth. It is instead a wonderful roller coaster of sweet and disorderly chaos and clutter, smiles and worry, battle cries and lullabies, ecstasy and wonderment, with constant overtones of hard work, busted budgets, and the glorious feeling that I have the privilege of influencing the life of another human being for good."

A MOTHER OF FOUR AND GRANDMOTHER OF TEN

"I am amazed at how many people stop me to have a look at my baby. Motherhood seems to break all social barriers as conversations with strangers of all ages and backgrounds evolve."

SIMONE BLOOM

"The entry of a child into any situation changes the whole situation."

I. MURDOCH

"God sends children for another purpose than merely
to keep up the race—to enlarge our hearts; to make us
unselfish and full of kindly sympathies and affections;
to give our souls higher aims and to call out all our
faculties; to extend enterprise and exertion; to bring
'round our firesides bright faces and happy smiles and
loving, tender hearts. My soul blesses the great Father
every day that He has gladdened the earth with little
children."

MARY HEWITT

"And there he was—a red-faced, black-haired,
frowning baby—a real person with hands and feet and
a real face. They whisked him away. Something was
real and alive inside that blue blanket I had bought so
casually in Macy's. A real creature, all mine."

DOROTHY EVSLIN

"The third baby is the easiest. You know, for instance,
how you're going to look in a maternity dress about
the seventh month, and you know how to release the
foot brake on a baby carriage without fumbling
amateurishly."

SHIRLEY JACKSON

"It wasn't a kick at all, which is what I had been led to
expect, but a flickering, like a little butterfly alive in my
belly."

SOPHIA LOREN

THINGS TO KNOW

In nine months, you will have come a long way, Mom. The staggering truth is that the size of a woman's uterus increases five hundred times before the birth of her baby.

Baby's movements, especially the first ones, are a confirmation that there truly is a new life growing in your womb. The exciting truth that you are creating a new life inside becomes real. Baby's jumping-jack tactics affirm what you have had to take someone else's word for, up to now.

When my baby moves, it feels like:

_____

_____

_____

_____

_____

_____

_____

_____

_____

_____

_____

When Baby sleeps, all is usually quiet inside. When Baby wakes, there is likely to be some stretching of legs and arms. So when Mom feels she is being jabbed by elbows or toes, she probably is. "Sleep time" is longer than "awake time." Some babies sleep with chin tucked under. Others sleep with their head back or to the side. Each seems to have a favorite position.

What I was doing when I first felt life inside:

_____

_____

_____

_____

_____

_____

_____

_____

_____

_____

_____

_____

_____

_____

Time to rejoice! Baby's kicking has made him or her become a rather uneasy rider inside you. Suddenly an experience that seemed unreal—even surreal—a pregnancy that was to be believed although it was neither seen nor felt becomes very real indeed. Baby is really in there. This sensational stirring inside the womb is often called "quickening." However, some women may say, "I have now felt 'life.'" In the early stages, Baby has lots of room for fetal aerobics. Movement resembles that of astronauts in a spaceship who float around the cabin in all directions.

My reaction when I first felt life was:

_____

_____

_____

_____

_____

_____

_____

_____

_____

_____

_____

Something from nothing!

Impossible, yet true!

He is the Creator.

Who else if not he?

*A*lmost every mother will tell you that when Baby arrives, her love for her child is far greater than she ever imagined. That love gives great motivation to do the best for the baby, and it is enough. You do not have to be someone who picks up every baby in sight and loves baby-sitting for every toddler in the neighborhood to catch on quickly to the important skills of parenting. Many, many women who have never thought much about babies at all or who have felt rather neutral about them or who have never even held a newborn become excellent mothers. It just works that way. So, take heart.

*W*hen the hospital nurse laid that precious, fragile package in my arms and said, "Goodbye and good luck," I felt alarmed. What did I know about babies? I wanted to go somewhere to take a college course in baby care, then be issued a diploma with a master's degree before journeying further into motherhood. After an anxious and uncertain week at home, a wise neighbor with three children told me, "Relax. Your baby won't break. But she can feel your nervousness. Just use common sense. Chances are you will do the right things." After that, I began to enjoy my new daughter. She became my friend. So did that wiser older woman.

Time with God

Place your hands on your belly and envision Baby curled up inside and aware of you as a friend, recognizing your voice, alert to your movement. Rejoice that you are creating. Now, close your eyes and imagine you are holding in your arms a new life, your own flesh, your own blood, that came from your own body. Do you sense the warmth of the tiny person wrapped in the soft blanket? Let your child grip a finger—feel it holding on tight? Now your baby is nuzzling at your breast, sharing the perfect sustaining elements that only you can give. Take heart, little mother. Motherhood is what your body was designed for.

Sure, pregnancy is difficult when you walk around with a big belly and bosom; when you feel like a ripe melon—full, fertile, and fat; when you have no waistline and can't even see your feet! The rest of the world seems to have an obsession with thinness and the beauty of a concave body. But rejoice, there is a live human being inside—a real person! Someone who will one day cry and talk and walk and love.

Focusing on the largeness of my pregnancy rather than on my large size, the huge miracle of it all, the majesty of creation and my baby's potential, helped me enjoy the added "girth of birth" and to see the real beauty in my convex shape. The pregnant body truly is extraordinarily beautiful because what it does is so incredible.

*T*ake a moment to imagine your baby growing inside—God himself reaching down hour by hour to create something out of nothing, new cells, new bone, new tissue, eyes, ears, nose, mouth, adding daily to your little one.

*H*ow precious are your thoughts about me, O God! They are innumerable! I can't even count them; they outnumber the grains of sand! And when I wake up in the morning, you are still with me!

PSALM 139:17-18, NLT

Prayer & Meditation

O God, the King of glory, you have exalted

your only Son Jesus Christ with great triumph

to your kingdom in heaven:

Do not leave us comfortless, but send us your

Holy Spirit to strengthen us, and exalt us to

that place where our Savior Christ has gone before;

who lives and reigns with you and the Holy Spirit,

one God, in glory everlasting.

BOOK OF COMMON PRAYER

Lord Jesus Christ, who dost embrace children with the arms of mercy . . . give (this child) grace . . . to stand fast in thy faith, to obey thy word, and to abide in thy love.

BOOK OF COMMON PRAYER

May the grace of Christ, our Savior,
And the Father's boundless love,
With the Holy Spirit's favor,
Rest upon us from above.

Thus may we abide in union
With each other and the Lord,
And possess, in sweet communion,
Joys which earth cannot afford.

The One Year Book of Hymns, SEPTEMBER 22

You who lie beneath my heart,
In whose soul I have no part;
Whose sweet shape will someday rest
Close, ah close! against my breast—
Breathe a prayer to God for me
That I love you worthily.

You whose eyes I have not seen,
Yet whose sight will be so keen
When you come to judge my life
With its foolishness and strife—
Breathe a prayer to God for me
That he give you Charity.

Anonymous

Dear Lord, I do not ask
That thou should'st give me some high work of thine,
Some noble calling, or some wond'rous task;
Give me a little hand to hold in mine,
Give me a little child to point the way
Over the strange, sweet path that leads to Thee:
Give me a little voice to teach to pray,
Give me two shining eyes Thy face to see.
The only crown I ask, dear Lord, to wear
Is this: that I may teach a little child.
I do not ask that I may ever stand
Among the wise, the worthy, or the great;
I only ask that softly, hand in hand,
A child and I may enter at the gate.

AUTHOR UNKNOWN

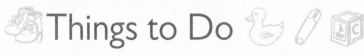# Things to Do

When visitors come, be sure to display and admire baby photos of the older youngster when you show first pictures of your newborn.

Things to do with older children: Make a mobile for Baby's room by punching holes in baby cards and hanging them from strings on a coat hanger above Baby's crib (hang firmly and well out of Baby's reach). The cards will move to entertain Baby and can be replaced as new ones arrive. Designs like stars or triangles, cut from plastic meat trays and hole-punched, make good additions to mobiles, too.

We forget that siblings, even young ones, often can be a real help for a tired mom. Kids love to feel needed, too. Ask for aid in setting the table, drying the silverware and putting it away, folding and sorting clothes, and dusting furniture. Post a list of tasks for teenagers who can drive, and assign them errands to the post office, library, or dentist

appointments with younger children. Maybe your teen will agree to be dropped off at the grocery store with a list while you are at the hairdresser or bank.

Buy a toy for Grandma's house every time you buy a new one for Baby. It won't take long to fill Grandma's toy chest, and baby-sitting will be a lot easier for her. When Baby Number Two comes along, toys will already be there.

Have a gala Grandma shower to celebrate this lady who gave birth to *you*, and invite your siblings to bring toys for her sitter's toy closet to be used whenever she baby-sits any other grandchildren too.

Have the house stocked ahead of time with groceries, cleaning items, and frozen foods. This will make life a little easier when you are away—and when the turmoil of Baby's first days at home takes over.

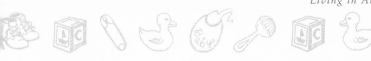

Buy two of everything to reduce shopping time spent.

One pregnant wife sensed that her husband felt a little left out of the baby shower joy. Her solution? She persuaded her mom and his mom to throw a dad-to-be shower. Gifts can include an alarm clock as a reminder of midnight feedings, a bird feeder to put outside the garage window, gardening tools, matching T-shirts for Mom and Dad, and favorite snacks. (How about one of the ten-pound chocolate bars available in bulk food stores?)

Changing smoke alarm batteries is a good way to prepare for your new baby. You will feel more at ease bringing an infant into the nursery knowing smoke detectors in your home are in good working order. Batteries should be changed twice a year according to fire-safety experts.

The last few weeks of pregnancy, clip baby-product coupons with long-term expiration dates for things like lotions, wipes, diapers, baby cereal, and so forth. You'll be glad you did when shower gifts run out and it is time to restock Baby's cupboard.

In the eighth or ninth month, it is a good idea to compile a list of helpful hints to make housekeeping easier for the family when you are away. Talk over child care arrangements with older youngsters so they will know what to expect. Write out names and phone numbers of folks for Dad to call after Baby arrives.

Many pregnant women prepare double batches of food during the last couple of months. These frozen meals can help Dad when he takes over the household and can ensure an easier homecoming for Mom and Baby.

Hang the most beautiful calendar you can find, preferably one with baby pictures, and make a big deal of having the family help you mark off the days remaining until Baby's "birth" day. Buy a special pen, maybe one that clicks to various colors, to be used only for the daily calendar countdown ritual. Begin about two months before Baby's due date.

While waiting for Baby, spend some time making a calendar with large spaces to write in brief descriptions of daily happenings after she arrives. Because you will hang the calendar near the changing table, it will be handier than running for the baby book all the time. Infants need changing frequently. Use this time to capture wonderful moments. You can write them down as they happen.

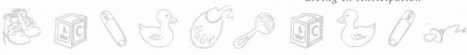

A baby's name is for a lifetime and often inspires images, both good and bad. It will be less often used by its owner than by others. Begin now to make a list of favorite names for both boys and girls. Say the names aloud and in combination with middle and last names to hear how they sound. Do names seem sensible for a grown-up as well as for someone in kindergarten? As the months go by, narrow the list to fifteen, then ten, then five by the final month so there will be no delay in filing Baby's birth certificate.

One clever grandma-to-be used her son's college sweatshirts to sew a patchwork quilt she called "Daddy's blanket." Made of heavy, flannel-backed material, it proved practical as a nice, soft floor blanket for Baby's play. Maybe all those T-shirt insignias you and Hubby have collected over the years from sports teams, concerts, and visits to exotic places could be cut and pieced together to make a memory quilt for Baby.

ALL

IN THE

FAMILY

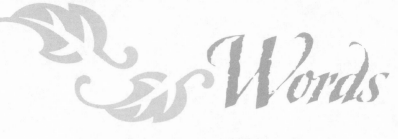

Words

Commit yourselves completely to these words of mine. Tie them to your hands as a reminder, and wear them on your forehead. Teach them to your children. Talk about them when you are at home and when you are away on a journey, when you are lying down and when you are getting up again. Write them on the doorposts of your house and on your gates, so that as long as the sky remains above the earth, you and your children may flourish. . . . Be careful to obey all the commands I give you; show love to the Lord your God by walking in his ways and clinging to him. The godly walk with integrity; blessed are their children after them.

DEUTERONOMY 11:18-22; PROVERBS 20:7, NLT

As for me and my family, we will serve the Lord.

JOSHUA 24:15, NLT

Who are those who fear the Lord? He will show them the path they should choose. They will live in prosperity, and their children will inherit the Promised Land.

PSALM 25:12-13, NLT

to Live By

The Lord is like a father to his children, tender and compassionate to those who fear him. For he understands how weak we are; he knows we are only dust. Our days on earth are like grass; like wildflowers, we bloom and die. But the love of the Lord remains forever with those who fear him. His salvation extends to the children's children of those who are faithful . . . who obey his commandments!

PSALM 103:13-18, NLT

*C*hildren are an heritage of the Lord: and the fruit of the womb is his reward. As arrows are in the hand of a mighty man; so are children of the youth. Happy is the man that hath his quiver full of them.

PSALM 127:3-5, KJV

*G*ood people leave an inheritance to their grandchildren, but the sinner's wealth passes to the godly.

PROVERBS 13:22, NLT

Those who fear the Lord are secure; he will be a place of refuge for their children.

PROVERBS 14:26, NLT

May the Lord of peace himself always give you his peace no matter what happens. The Lord be with you all.

2 THESSALONIANS 3:16, NLT

I know that you sincerely trust the Lord, for you have the faith of your mother, Eunice, and your grandmother, Lois. This is why I remind you to fan into flames the spiritual gift God gave you when I laid my hands on you.

2 TIMOTHY 1:5-6, NLT

A word for dads and moms from the heavenly Father:

Love each other with true Christian love. Give honor to marriage, and remain faithful to one another. Each man must love his wife as he loves himself, and the wife must respect her husband.

HEBREWS 13:1, 4; EPHESIANS 5:33, NLT

Scripture help for parents:

Be sympathetic, love . . . be compassionate and humble. Do not repay evil with evil or insult with insult, but with blessing, because to this you were called so that you may inherit a blessing. . . . "Keep [your] tongue from evil and [your] lips from deceitful speech. . . . Turn from evil and do good; . . . seek peace and pursue it. For the eyes of the Lord are on the righteous and his ears are attentive to their prayer, but the face of the Lord is against those who do evil." . . . If you should suffer for what is right, you are blessed.

1 PETER 3:8-14, NIV

Those who live in the shelter of the Most High will find rest in the shadow of the Almighty. This I declare of the Lord: He alone is my refuge, my place of safety; he is my God, and I am trusting him.

PSALM 91:1-2, NLT

Go home to your friends, and tell them what wonderful things the Lord has done for you and how merciful he has been.

MARK 5:19, NLT

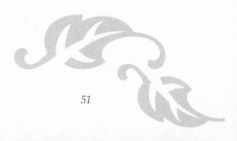

"Worth Repeating"

"One thing so simple a child can operate is a grandmother [or grandfather]."

"More children are spoiled because the parents won't spank Grandma."

"Grandparents are baby-sitters who watch the baby instead of TV."

"The advantage of a large family is that at least one of the children may not turn out like the others."

"The best thing a man can do for his children is to love their mother."

"I always think that in the end children educate their parents."

PRINCESS ALICE

"It's not easy being a mother. If it were, fathers would do it."

DOROTHY, *The Golden Girls*

"A family is . . . a unit composed not only of children, but of men, women, an occasional animal, and the common cold."

OGDEN NASH

"A newborn is merely a small, noisy object, slightly
fuzzy at one end, with no distinguishing marks to
speak of except a mouth. But to its immediate family it
is without question the most phenomenal, the most
astonishing, the most absolutely unparalleled thing
that has yet occurred in the entire history of this
planet."

IRVING COBB

"Child of my heart, lying under my heart, with my
relationship to you has grown a new relationship to
your father; he is more than lover, husband, and king.
. . . Love has become sacred and holy beyond words,
almost beyond thought."

ELLIS MEREDITH

"When grandchildren visit their grandparents, it is the
happiest day in the grandparents' lives. The only day
that is happier is when they go home."

SIR FREDERICK MESSER

"If you're having your first baby, make sure you get a
grandmother there as soon as possible. You may think
you know all there is to know about life, but you can't
touch her when it comes to this."

BOB GREENE

"Nobody asked me if I wanted a little sister."

GALE LYNN, AGE FOUR

THINGS TO KNOW

More than ten thousand babies are born daily in the United States.

Rosanna Della Corta of Viterbo, Italy is believed to be the oldest mother in the world. She was sixty-two years old when her child was born.

Each year, about 175,000 babies are born to dads who are at least forty years old. At the same time, 31,000 are born to mothers who are at least forty years old.

DANIEL E. WEISS

Never again in his life, in so brief a period, will this human being grow so rapidly or so much, or develop in so many directions, as he does between conception and birth. During this critical period, the development of the human body exhibits the most perfect time and the most elaborate correlations that we ever display in our entire lives. The building and launching of a satellite, involving thousands of people and hundreds of electronic devices, is not nearly so complex an operation as the building and launching of a human being.

ASHLEY MONTAGUE, ANTRHROPOLOGIST

The history of man

for the nine months preceding his birth

would probably be far more interesting,

and contain events of greater moment,

than all the threescore and ten years

that follow it.

SAMUEL TAYLOR COLERIDGE

Are you taking time to revel in your personal miracle of mother-hood? Set aside a few minutes daily to quietly relish the fascinating fact that you are creating a new life, another complex body, within yourself. Purposefully nurture positive feelings about this amazing body of yours. You can go to work, carry on a conversation, make love, shower, take care of other children, and do hundreds of additional things—all while carrying out the enormously complex task of growing a new person within your belly. You yourself are a miracle! Have fun dressing, and enjoy the way you look with your baby inside. Remind yourself that one person is becoming two.

The baby is closely confined in a warm, dark prison of exquisite, neutral comfort. Everything around him is of the same texture and at the same temperature as himself. Amniotic fluid fills the spaces between his body and the walls of the womb; there is no friction. . . . His eyes are ready but there is nothing for him to see. He has no need to breathe nor does he need to digest food. . . . He can sense sound and movement, but even they are muffled by his insulated liquid environment. He is sealed off from the world, untouched and untouchable.

PENELOPE LEACH

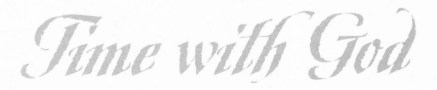

Time with God

At this very moment, thousands of women around the world are having babies. I am not isolated in carrying and delivering mine. When I think about all those other mothers' children who were birthed in bygone eras in exactly the same way—millions, no, billions of them—the process of labor and delivery seems less threatening, perfectly normal. It might be new to me, but it has been going on since the beginning of time. I am part of a vibrant chain of life that has existed since Adam and Eve and has involved women from times and countries long forgotten, both primitive and civilized—nomadic women, Stone and Bronze Age women, Bible women, wealthy wives of presidents, and the humble wives of their servants. Every baby had an impact, small or large, on history. Mine will too.

Let us . . . lay aside every weight and sin that clings so closely, and let us run with perseverance the race that is set before us, looking to Jesus the pioneer and perfecter of our faith.

HEBREWS 12:1-2, NRSV

Some babies suck their thumbs incessantly in the womb. No one really knows why. It has been reported that a few are even born with calluses on their thumbs!

"My Thumb, My Treasure"
If a babe suck his thumb
'Tis an ease to his gum;
A comfort, a boon,
A calmer of grief,
A friend in his need affording relief;
A solace, a good,
A soother of pain,
A composer to sleep
A charm and a gain.

ANONYMOUS

Prayer & Meditation

Savior, like a shepherd lead us,

Much we need Thy tender care;

In thy pleasant pastures feed us,

For our use Thy folds prepare;

Blessed Jesus, blessed Jesus!

Thou has bought us, Thine we are.

The One Year Book of Hymns, SEPTEMBER 24

The responsibilities of fatherhood often drive us to our knees. So many things regarding our families are beyond our control, we need to enlist the power of God to accomplish what we cannot do.

The patriarchs of Israel—Abraham, Isaac, and Jacob—were praying fathers, as were Moses and Joshua. The great walled city of Jericho seemed impregnable, but Joshua's obedient faith brought the walls down. This prayerful leader left a statement of faith that removes all doubt about his confidence in God to answer his prayers for his family. "As for me and my house, we will serve the Lord" (Joshua 24:15, KJV).

ROGER CAMPBELL

Write here your prayer for Baby's dad:

_____

_____

_____

Celebrate Thanksgiving in any month of the year: Ask the kids to help you plan a "Thank you, God, for our new baby" family celebration after Mom and Baby have had a chance to get used to each other and the household has developed a more relaxed routine. Maybe Dad or one of the older children can read some praise verses from the Psalms. Small children can help light candles and offer thank-you prayers.

Write a prayer asking God to make love your greatest aim:

_____

_____

_____

_____

Write a prayer asking God to make love the greatest aim of Baby's father:

_____

_____

_____

_____

Write a love letter to Baby's father.

_____

_____

_____

_____

_____

Unless the Lord builds a house, the work of the builders is useless.

PSALM 127:1, NLT

O God, the protector of all who trust in you, without whom nothing is strong, nothing is holy: Increase and multiply upon us your mercy . . . you as our ruler and guide.

BOOK OF COMMON PRAYER

Things to Do

Your doctor will very likely be interested in Baby's father too, especially his health history. If possible, Dad and Mom should go together on one of the first visits to the obstetrician's office.

If Dad's job will be to watch out for an older sibling after Baby arrives, remind him that his young charge will greatly need the extra attention with so much focused on Baby. Suggest he try to convey to the youngster that this will be a good chance for the two of them to spend fun time together.

To get Baby off to a good start with siblings, plan ahead for Dad or someone else to carry the newborn into the house when you return from the hospital so you can devote complete attention to the other children for the first few minutes.

Have wrapped surprises on hand for Baby's siblings so they won't feel left out when gifts arrive for your newcomer.

If your doctor prescribes an ultrasound, ask Dad to videotape it, then invite aunts, uncles, and grandparents to see the exciting images. Keep the picture of the ultrasound. Later, when you assemble a collection of Baby's photos, you'll have the ultrasound as the very first one.

Check out your local hospital or birthing center to see if sibling-orientation classes are offered. Many mothers-to-be think the classes offer terrific ideas for use in helping older children adjust more easily when the newborn arrives to share home and attention.

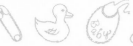

A young child will enjoy touring the hospital or birthing center. Let her help pick a gift for Baby from the gift shop and maybe a toy for herself. Visit the nursery if permitted. Your youngster will know where you will be the first day or two after Baby arrives. Make sure she knows you will be returning home after a short time. Or take children to visit a friend with a new baby so they can get an idea what newborns are like.

It may be exciting for extended family members or Baby's siblings to go with you for a doctor visit to listen to Baby's heartbeat.

To help young children feel they are really a part of this "new baby" process, talk with them at quiet moments about your pregnancy. Allow tummy patting, share thoughts and feelings, and let them talk to the new baby inside using your belly button as a microphone.

Ask youngsters what they think it is like to live in such a small space. Borrow children's library books to read together about newborns.

Sitters can be fun: There will be fewer tears when the sitter arrives if you let the child know that there will be special, fun activities to do. Young children enjoy baking with an adult, learning to knit on extra-large needles, pasting magazine cutouts into a book, stuffing a doll, or listening to a favorite story.

Bedtime may be the most difficult time. A taped message of reassurance, fun, love, or a lullaby sung in your familiar voice and played just before being tucked in could be a real comfort. Or, tape a favorite story, tell a secret, or promise something the two of you will be doing together when you return.

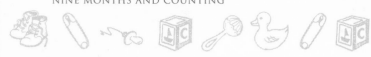

Photo: Leaving a photograph of yourself on your child's dresser will let him know you care. Be sure to give assurance that you definitely will return home. Or, leave a surprise note under the pillow.

Daily presents: Let the child see a small tote bag full of wrapped gifts you will be leaving for him to open every few hours while you are away.

Together though apart: Agree on a favorite mystery story, book, or Bible chapters for both you and your child to read while apart (the sitter will read to young children). Having something in common to talk about on the phone or when you return will add a bit of togetherness. One mother gave her fourth grader a new diary because "I will miss a part of your life while I'm gone, and we can share together what you write when I return."

Long-distance fun: If you will be gone for an extended period of time, as for a cesarean, call your child daily, or have Dad bring home small gifts from the hospital, things like plastic medicine cups, flexi-straws, or a pudding cup from your dinner tray.

Simple baby-care tasks can be assigned to siblings after the newborn arrives home, things like folding and piling diapers and baby clothing, bringing items to Mom while she is feeding Baby, keeping baby articles neat on the shelf by the changing table. Let youngsters know how much their help is needed and appreciated so they can feel a part of this new area of family life.

To keep siblings occupied while you feed Baby, place a basket near your chair that is filled with playthings—games that can be played alone, coloring books and crayons, puzzles, a tape player with

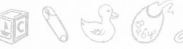

headphones, and picture books. These will be used only while Mom is feeding Baby.

Leave articles to take along (things like returns to stores, dry cleaning, clothes for alteration and packages to be mailed) in one place near the door so they are ready when you are and you won't need to search for them.

Save bank trips by arranging for direct deposit, then pay bills by mail. Pool errands with coworkers or neighbors so they can share some of the running around.

Set limits on your workload, then ask for help from someone around you if you are stressed out. Being direct has the best chance: "Would you please consider getting supper for five nights? I really need some time in the day to be by myself." Many women never think to ask so forthrightly. Hinting and

complaining will probably get you nowhere.

Always park near the same place in parking lots so you won't be hunting down your car. Take along a list of errands to be done in sequence, so you won't be backtracking and wasting time and energy.

FACING

ANXIETY

Words

This is the history of the family of Isaac, the son of Abraham. When Isaac was forty years old, he married Rebekah. . . . Isaac pleaded with the Lord to give Rebekah a child because she was childless. So the Lord answered Isaac's prayer, and his wife became pregnant with twins [Esau and Jacob]. But the two children struggled with each other in her womb. So she went to ask the Lord about it. . . . The Lord told her, "The sons in your womb will become two rival nations. One nation will be stronger than the other; the descendants of your older son will serve the descendants of your younger son." Isaac was sixty years old when the twins were born.

GENESIS 25:19-23, 26, NLT

Rachel's story: Jacob was tricked into thinking he would be rewarded with Rachel as his bride after seven years of work. Instead, he was given Leah, who was not his real love, and he had to work another seven years to be given Rachel.

to Live By

Because Leah was unloved, the Lord let her have a child, while Rachel was childless. When Rachel saw that she wasn't having any children, she became jealous of her sister. "Give me children, or I'll die!" she exclaimed to Jacob. Jacob flew into a rage. "Am I God?" he asked. "He is the only one able to give you children."

Then Rachel told him, "Sleep with my servant, Bilhah [a common practice of the day], and she will bear children for me." Bilhah became pregnant and presented him with a son. [Leah also gave birth to her fifth son and a daughter.]

[Later:] God remembered Rachel's plight and answered her prayers by giving her a child . . . a son. "God has removed my shame," she said. And she named him Joseph.

GENESIS 29–30, NLT, SELECTED

The story of Abraham and Sarah:

Abram replied, "O Sovereign Lord, what good are all your blessings when I don't even have a son?. . . You have given me no children, so one of my servants will have to be my heir." Then the Lord said to him, "No, your servant will not be your heir, for you will have a son of your own to inherit everything I am giving you."

GENESIS 15:2-4, NLT

Sarai, Abram's wife, had no children. So Sarai took her servant, an Egyptian woman named Hagar, and gave her to Abram so she could bear his children. "The Lord has kept me from having any children," Sarai said to Abram. "Go and sleep with my servant. Perhaps I can have children through her. . . ."

Abram slept with Hagar, and she became pregnant. When Hagar knew she was pregnant, she began to treat her mistress Sarai with contempt. Then Sarai said to Abram, "It's all your fault! Now this servant of mine is pregnant, and she despises me. . . . The Lord will make you pay for doing this to me!" Abram replied, "Since she is your servant, you may deal with her as you see fit." So Sarai treated her harshly, and Hagar ran away. . . .

Then the angel of the Lord said [to Hagar], "Return to your mistress and submit to her authority. . . . You are now pregnant and will give birth to a son. You are to name him Ishmael. . . . This son of yours will be a wild one—free and untamed as a wild donkey! He will be against everyone, and everyone will be against him. Yes, he will live at odds with the rest of his brothers. . . ." So Hagar gave Abram a son, and Abram named him Ishmael. Abram was eighty-six years old at that time.

Genesis 16:1-15, NLT, selected

The story continues:

When Abram was ninety-nine years old, the Lord appeared to him and said, "I am God Almighty. . . . I will make you the father of not just one nation, but a multitude of nations! What's more, I am changing your name. . . . Now you will be known as Abraham. . . . I will give you millions of descendants. . . . Regarding Sarai, your wife—her name will no longer be Sarai; from now on you will call her Sarah. And I will bless her and give you a son from her!"

Genesis 17:1-6, 15-16, NLT

Woe to you who strive with your Maker, earthen vessels with the potter! Does the clay say to the one who fashions it, "What are you making"? or "Your work has no handles"? Woe to anyone who says to a father, "What are you begetting?" or to a woman, "With what are you in labor?" Thus says the Lord, the Holy One . . . : Will you question me . . . or command me concerning the work of my hands?

Isaiah 45:9-11, NRSV

He will feed his flock like a shepherd. He will carry the lambs in his arms, holding them close to his heart. He will gently lead the mother sheep with their young.

ISAIAH 40:11, NLT

Lord, you are our Father. We are the clay, and you are the potter. We are all formed by your hand.

ISAIAH 64:8, NLT

He is the God who made the world and everything in it. . . . He himself gives life and breath to everything. . . . After all, we didn't bring anything with us when we came into the world, and we certainly cannot carry anything with us when we die.

ACTS 17:24-25; 1 TIMOTHY 6:6-7, NLT

We grow weary in our present bodies, and we long for the day when we will put on our heavenly bodies like new clothing. Our aim is to please him always.

2 CORINTHIANS 5:2, 9, NLT

Ye are of God, little children. . . . Greater is he that is in you, than he that is in the world.

1 JOHN 4:4, KJV

*R*emember the Sabbath day by keeping it holy. Six days
you shall labor and do all your work, but the seventh day
is a Sabbath to the Lord your God. . . . In six days the
Lord made the heavens and the earth, the sea, and all that
is in them, but he rested on the seventh day.

Exodus 20:8-11, NIV

"Worth Repeating"

"When doubts take over, remember that there is wonderful joy ahead when life with Baby becomes more routine, more comfortable."

"Of all our infirmities, the most savage is to despise our being."

MONTAIGNE

"Behind the dim unknown, standeth God within the shadow, keeping watch above his own."

ROBERT LOWELL

"Quiet minds cannot be perplexed or frightened, but go on in fortune or misfortune at their own private pace, like the ticking of a clock during a thunderstorm."

ROBERT LOUIS STEVENSON

"No job on earth takes more physical, mental, social, emotional and spiritual strength than being a good wife and mother. If a gal's looking for the easy life, she might try teaching tennis, cutting diamonds, or joining a Roller Derby team. There is nothing easy about good mothering. It can be backbreaking, heart wrenching, and anxiety producing. And that's just the morning."

STEVEN AND JANET BLY

"There are some days, which to have lived through is
   to have done more than one's duty!"

MARION VAN HORNE

"I actually remember feeling delight at two o'clock in
   the morning when the baby woke for his feed because I
   so longed to have another look at him."

MARGARET DRABBLE

"Let nothing disturb thee,
   Nothing affright thee;
   All things are passing;
   God never changeth;
   Patient endurance
   Attaineth to all things;
   Who God possesseth
   In nothing is wanting;
   Alone God sufficeth."

ST. TERESA OF AVILA

"Fill your mind with the thought that God is there.
   And once your mind is truly filled with that thought,
   when you experience difficulties it will be as easy as
   breathing for you to remember, my heavenly Father
   knows all about this! Therefore, you can rest in perfect
   confidence in Him."

OSWALD CHAMBERS

The book of Jeremiah uses the words

"the Lord Almighty" seventy-six times.

If my faith is wavering,

it is being shaped by something other than the

all-powerful God who is Lord of hosts—

thousands and thousands of angels, stars, and earth.

When I dwell on the negative things in my life, I forget my Father's power.

What is my perception of God and his care? Are my circumstances a barrier to believing that nothing is too difficult for him?

It is somehow in God's plan that he wants to hear us voice our wishes. Surely God delights in being able to give good gifts to his children, gifts for which they have asked. It is something like a youngster who, at Christmas, expresses a desire for a certain toy. What parent has not experienced delight in being able to grant that wish? Yet, when a good parent says no, that is for the best. God is like that too.

Don't you know that the Lord is the everlasting God, the Creator of all the earth? He never grows faint or weary. . . . He gives power to those who are tired and worn out; he offers strength to the weak. Those who wait on the Lord will find new strength. They will fly high on wings like eagles. They will run and not grow weary. They will walk and not faint.

ISAIAH 40:28-29, 31, NLT

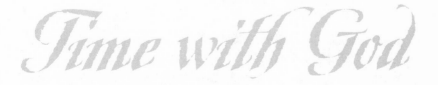

There is an unhurried flow of power available to us who belong to God. Have you forgotten?

Doctors say some depressed feelings are normal during pregnancy. Purposely replacing fearful or negative thoughts with more positive thinking is a biblical concept. To help yourself, make a list of twenty-five positive things that are going on in your life. Whistle! Sing aloud! Read the words of uplifting hymns. Memorize some of the Scriptures in this book.

Today I will meditate on God's wonderful miracles in making the world and on how he has brought me this far in life. I will meditate on Andrew Murray's description of the joy that lies ahead: "There is perhaps no such moment of exquisite joy, of deep, unutterable thanksgiving taking the place of pain and sorrow, as when a woman knows herself to be the living mother of a living child."

Today, I will remember that it is OK to feel God's relaxation and peace even if there are lots of problems everywhere. It is OK to breathe deeply and feel serene, then breathe deeply again and gain more serenity. Peace is for everyone. God never meant for me to feel anxious or down so much of the time.

Imagine God walking beside you (and your baby), holding your hand, all day long today.

These are the most common concerns of a pregnant woman: Will my baby be normal? Will I somehow lose my baby in miscarriage? Should I quit my job and stay home to care for Baby? How will we manage financially? If I stay home with Baby, will I feel cheated or dissatisfied or bored? With my body growing and changing, am I still appealing to my partner? The pain of labor worries me. Can I really be a good parent?

You are not alone in your concerns. This very moment, thousands upon thousands of others are carrying babies and having similar thoughts. Women have been handling childbirth in both the good and bad places very ably since the beginning of time. Most importantly, we do not stand alone in this world—God is our helper.

Pregnant women who encounter sluggish feelings find themselves in a dilemma trying to carry out the responsibilities of busy lives. New mothers do, too. If you feel intense fatigue before Baby is born or after, you are not alone. Almost all mothers and mothers-to-be complain of tiredness at one time or another. Think about this: just before Baby comes, Mom is usually carrying around twenty-five to thirty pounds of added weight, maybe more! Afterward, there are many adjustments to be made that can easily overwhelm anybody. Pregnancy and motherhood both bring a variety of symptoms, most unavoidable and, fortunately, temporary. Our own strength is insufficient.

Prayer & Meditation

Lord, just now, help me to feel your great love

like beautiful warm sunshine flowing over me.

I open my mind to let your love take over.

Help me to lose in that flow of love all my doubts,

all my fears, and all my anxieties about becoming a mother.

Take away my tensions and turmoil.

Replace negative and pessimistic thoughts

with a brand-new confident spirit

that fills my anxious mind with excitement, meaning, and delight.

Make parenting a tremendous experience, instead of a fearsome one.

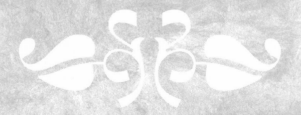

Lord, the state of the world is so upsetting today; nothing seems secure or sure because everything is changing fast. Some of the drift is frightening, far, far removed from what I thought you planned. New things are terribly complicated. Crime and rebellion and war and deadly earthquakes and floods are headlined daily. Sometimes I feel lost and alone and confused. Please, Lord, fix the great truths of Scripture in my mind so my heart becomes confident about my future and my baby's. You never change, and you are always nearby to help and to love us. Keep me walking the road following close behind you. I want to trust you to guide me.

My soul trusteth in thee: yea, in the shadow of thy wings will I make

my refuge. . . . I will cry unto God most high; unto God that

performeth all things for me. . . . God shall send forth his mercy. . . .

Be thou exalted, O God, above the heavens; let thy glory be above all

the earth. My heart is fixed, O God, my heart is fixed.

PSALM 57:1-3, 5, 7, KJV

Search me, O God, and know my heart; try me, and know my

thoughts: And see if there be any wicked way in me, and lead me in

the way everlasting.

PSALM 139:23-24, KJV

Under His wings I am safely abiding;
Though the night deepens and tempests are wild,
Still I can trust Him? I know He will keep me;
He has redeemed me and I am His child.

Under His wings, under His wings,
Who from His love can sever?
Under His wings my soul shall abide,
Safely abide forever.

The One Year Book of Hymns, OCTOBER 19

The Holy Spirit helps us in our distress.
For we don't even know what we should pray for,
nor how we should pray.
But the Holy Spirit prays for us with groanings
that cannot be expressed in words.

ROMANS 8:26, NLT

Create in me a pure heart, O God,

and renew a steadfast spirit within me.

PSALM 51:10, NIV

Don't worry about anything; instead, pray about everything.

Tell God what you need, and thank him for all he has done.

If you do this, you will experience God's peace,

which is far more wonderful than the human mind can understand.

His peace will guard your hearts and minds

as you live in Christ Jesus.

PHILIPPIANS 4:6-7, NLT

Give thanks for the Lord's ability

to grant peace and freedom from fear.

Help me to do the very best I can to bring up my baby as Scripture instructs: "Whatsoever thy hand findeth to do, do it with thy might" (Ecclesiastes 9:10, KJV).

Write here a prayer telling God your personal needs:

_____

_____

_____

List your fears:

_____

_____

_____

Give them over to God right now. Are there troubles you have dragged along in your life from day to day? Read Job 36–39 and Job 42:2, then ask yourself, "Is there anything at all that the God who made and governs the universe cannot handle?"

Realize that God is not the source of worry. When worry comes, say aloud, "Stop." Then purposely but gently move your mind and thoughts over to another subject. If worry returns, repeat this peaceful process.

When your mind is troubled, repeat Philippians 4:6-7 aloud as many times as it takes to clear away worries. Memorize it and write it here:

_____

_____

_____

_____

FINDING

ASSURANCE

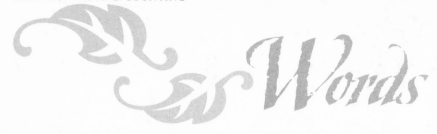

Words

Scripture blessing on the new mother:

The Lord bless thee, and keep thee: The Lord make his face shine upon thee, and be gracious unto thee: The Lord lift up his countenance upon thee, and give thee peace.

NUMBERS 6:24-26, KJV

Our help is in the name of the Lord, who made heaven and earth.

PSALM 124:8, KJV

To remember in times of worry and stress:

From birth I have relied on you; you brought me forth from my mother's womb. I will ever praise you.

PSALM 71:6, NIV

to Live By

I don't concern myself with matters too great or awesome for me. But I have stilled and quieted myself, just as a small child is quiet with its mother. The Lord God is my strength and my song; he has become my salvation.

PSALM 131:1-2; ISAIAH 12:2, NLT

Those who are wise will take all this to heart; they will see in our history the faithful love of the Lord.

PSALM 107:43, NLT

As one whom his mother comforteth, so will I comfort you.

ISAIAH 66:13, KJV

Be strong and courageous! Do not be afraid or discouraged. Give your burdens to the Lord, and he will take care of you.

JOSHUA 1:9; PSALM 55:22, NLT

God knows about pregnancy, labor, and birth. He labored over the birth of his beloved Israel for forty years from its beginning at Sinai. He himself conceived the nation of Israel, delivered her from the hand of Pharaoh, and brought her forth into new life in the Promised Land.

Has a nation ever been born in a single day? Has a country ever come forth in a mere moment? . . . Would I ever bring this nation to the point of birth and then not deliver it?" asks the Lord. "No! I would never keep this nation from being born."

ISAIAH 66:8-9, NLT

Not even a sparrow, worth only half a penny, can fall to the ground without your Father knowing it. And the very hairs on your head [Baby's too!] are all numbered. So don't be afraid; you are more valuable to him than a whole flock of sparrows.

MATTHEW 10:29-31, NLT

I pray that you will begin to understand the incredible greatness of his power for us who believe him. This is the same mighty power that raised Christ from the dead and seated him in the place of honor at God's right hand in the heavenly realms.

EPHESIANS 1:19-20, NLT

May our Lord Jesus Christ and God our Father, who loved us and in his special favor gave us everlasting comfort and good hope, comfort your hearts and give you strength in every good thing you do and say.

2 THESSALONIANS 2:16, NLT

But Christ, the faithful Son, was in charge of the entire household. And we are God's household.

HEBREWS 3:6, NLT

You will have courage because you will have hope.

JOB 11:18, NLT

I lie awake thinking of you, meditating on you through the night. I think how much you have helped me; I sing for joy in the shadow of your protecting wings. I follow close behind you; your strong right hand holds me securely.

PSALM 63:6-8, NLT

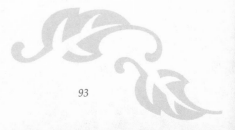

I cry out to God Most High. He will send help from heaven. My heart is confident in you, O God. For your unfailing love is as high as the heavens.

PSALM 57:2, 3, 7, 10, NLT

Whom have I in heaven but you? I desire you more than anything on earth. My health may fail, and my spirit may grow weak, but God remains the strength of my heart; he is mine forever.

PSALM 73:25-26, NLT

The Lord lifts up those who are bowed down, the Lord loves the righteous. The Lord . . . sustains the fatherless and the widow.

PSALM 146:8-9, NIV

For you are my hiding place; you protect me from trouble. You surround me with songs of victory. Interlude The Lord says, "I will guide you along the best pathway for your life. I will advise you and watch over you."

PSALM 32:7-8, NLT

If you make the Lord your refuge, if you make the Most High your shelter, . . . he orders his angels to protect you wherever you go. They will hold you with their hands to keep you. . . .

PSALM 91:9, 11-12, NLT

For God has not given us a spirit of fear and timidity, but of power, love, and self-discipline.

2 TIMOTHY 1:7, NLT

A glad heart makes a happy face.

PROVERBS 15:13, NLT

The race is not to the swift or the battle to the strong.

ECCLESIASTES 9:11, NIV

My grace is sufficient for you, for power is made perfect in weakness.

2 CORINTHIANS 12:9, NRSV

"Worth Repeating"

"Christ be with me, Christ within me,
Christ behind me, Christ before me,
Christ beside me, Christ to win me,
Christ to comfort me and restore me.
Christ beneath me, Christ above me.
Christ in quiet, Christ in danger,
Christ in hearts of all who love me,
Christ in mouth of friend or stranger."

ST. PATRICK

"God made mothers before he made ministers: the progress of Christ's kingdom depends more upon the influence of faithful, wise and pious mothers than upon any other human agency."

T. L. CUYLER

"The mother's love is like God's love: He loves us not because we are lovable, but because it is his nature to love, and because we are his children."

EARL RINEY

"When I stopped seeing my mother with the eyes of a child, I saw the woman who helped me give birth to myself."

NANCY FRIDAY

"I came home from the doctor's visit knowing I had gained five pounds in the seventh month. My mirror told clearly the story of my body's incredibly large size. I felt clumsy and ugly when I looked through a women's magazine featuring svelte models with perfect hairdos, slim bodies and beautiful formfitting clothes.

That all changed when my husband came home. Strangely, he seemed to love me more. He took me and our unborn child in his arms to be loved and hugged, and we kissed and kissed some more. The three of us love each other, he said. Suddenly we were a family, complete, just the way the Lord planned it. The family is a wonderful thing."

NEW YORK MOTHER-TO-BE

"You are free only when you can accept the past for what it is and only when you can accept your parents for who they are. And let it be. Then take up responsibility for your own present."

MARK TROTTER

"Certainly the world owes more to the prayers of women than it realizes."

HERBERT LOCKYER

"No man is poor who had a godly mother."

ABRAHAM LINCOLN

"Hidden in the hollow of His blessed hand,
Never foe can follow, never traitor stand;
Not a surge of worry, not a shade of care,
Not a blast of hurry touch the spirit there.
Stayed upon Jehovah, hearts are truly blest,
Finding as he promised, perfect peace and rest."

FRANCES R. HAVERGAL, "LIKE A RIVER GLORIOUS"

"Put everything in your life afloat upon God, going out
to sea on the great swelling tide of His purpose, and
your eyes will be opened. If you believe in Jesus, you
are not to spend all your time in the calm waters just
inside the harbor, full of joy, but always tied to the
dock. You have to get out past the harbor into the great
depths of God, and begin to know things for
yourself—begin to have spiritual discernment."

OSWALD CHAMBERS

"We must not get so busy counting demons that we
forget the holy angels. Certainly we are up against a
gigantic war machine. But we are encompassed by a
heavenly host so powerful that we need not fear the
warfare—the battle is the Lord's. If your valley is full of
foes, raise your sights to the hills and see the holy
angels of God arrayed for battle in your behalf. God
has promised in Hebrews 1:14: "Are they [angels] not
all ministering spirits, sent forth to minister for them
who shall be heirs of salvation?"

BILLY GRAHAM, *Angels*

"It was many years after I left the parental roof before I
came to the knowledge of salvation by faith in Christ.
But during all those years of wandering I never got
beyond the reach of my mother's prayers. Again and
again when Satan tempted me and sin allured me,
there rose up before me the vision of a little woman in
a checkered apron kneeling at that bed in the humble
home in western Michigan, and I heard her earnest
pleading with God for the salvation of her children as
she called them all by name, one by one, and claimed
them all for Christ. The memory of my name in
Mother's prayer had more to do with my salvation,
next to God Himself, than any other thing in the
world."

DR. M. R. DeHAAN

Someone has said that an infant in its mother's

womb feels the rhythm of her steps and is comforted

by the beating of her warm heart for nine months.

God knows the rhythm of my walking and my heart

thoughts too. He is as close as breathing as I live

through these nine months with my baby inside.

The sun stood still. The iron did swim.
This God is our God for ever and ever.
He will be our guide unto death.

Unknown

*If my God can make babies, walk on the water, heal the blind and
sick, and create the world and universe out of nothing by merely
saying a word, if he knows the number of hairs on my head and
counts the stars, calling them all by name—as Scripture says—then
surely I can trust him in all matters.*

God is much more committed to me than I am to him.
For this I am grateful.

*Jesus will give vitality and energy and life. Look to him for it. Ask
him for it. Then, don't forget to claim it.*

*Consider the farmers who eagerly look for the rains in the fall and
in the spring. They patiently wait for the precious harvest of grain,
vegetables, and fruit to ripen. You, too, must be patient. The fruit you
bring forth is far more valuable and even bears God's image.*

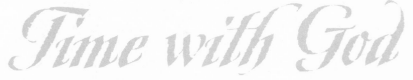

Time with God

Lord, what a master designer you are! My enlarged belly is the perfectly protected place for you to shelter my baby snugly, safely, happily, and warmly. You can be depended on to respond and bring her forth into the world at just the right time. Where there is a design, there must be a designer. You, Lord, are that designer.

He is the God who made the world and everything in it. . . . He himself gives life and breath to everything.

Acts 17:24-25, NLT

God does not grow tired. When your energy runs out, when weariness sets in, go back to him anytime, day or night, and claim his strength. God created your body. He knows well how to re-create it with strength and vitality.

Today, in every menial task, envision yourself serving with the strength God provides. See him working, speaking, thinking through you.

Set aside time today for listening to beautiful and quiet music to relax you. Baby can hear the tranquil and calming sounds, too.

Set aside time today to watch a funny video or read a humorous book that will make you laugh. Laughter is relaxing and healing to the soul. Maybe Baby's too.

Set aside time today to go by yourself and relax by listening to the sounds of calmness. You will be surprised by the muted and often pleasant sounds missed in life's daily hustle and bustle—the singing of birds, the giggling and laughter of children, the comfort of a quietly ticking clock—and more.

Prayer & Meditation

Lord, sometimes I hate the enormity
of my body, my roundness.
Yet your Word says that "thou hast created all things" (Revelation 4:11, KJV)
and that "[you have] made everything beautiful
for its own time" (Ecclesiastes 3:11, NLT).
But sometimes it seems all that I am is my bulging belly.
It is what everybody sees and talks about when we meet.
I am defined as pregnant. Now, while the focus on Baby
is so intense, it is easy for everyone (me included)
to forget that there is much more to me than this
nine-month body project in which I am involved.
It helps to remind myself often that I am much more than
a mother-to-be. I am a person with talents, abilities,
hopes, ambitions, fears, longings, and passions.
I am somebody's daughter, wife, and much more.

Lord, after Baby arrives and life becomes more ordinary,

the person you and I know I really am will once again

be more apparent. Meanwhile, I am glad you

know me so well and love me just as I am.

Confirm [my] joy by a lively sense of your presence with [me],

and give [me] calm strength and patient wisdom as [I] seek to

bring this child to love all that is true and noble, just and pure,

lovable and gracious, excellent and admirable, following

the example of our Lord and Savior, Jesus Christ.

BOOK OF COMMON PRAYER

Grant us, O Lord, the blessing of those whose minds are stayed upon thee, so that we may be kept in perfect peace—a peace which cannot be broken. Let not our minds rest upon any creature, but only in the Creator; not upon goods, things, houses, lands, inventions of vanities or foolish fashions, lest our peace being broken, we become cross and brittle and given over to envy. From all such deliver us, O God, and grant us thy peace.

GEORGE FOX

Write here your praise prayer to God for bringing you and Baby safely this far through pregnancy. Include specific things for which you are grateful.

_____

_____

_____

_____

_____

_____

Well does the hymn put it: "Thou art coming to a King; large petitions with thee bring." We do not come to the back door of the house of mercy to receive the broken scraps . . . nor to eat the crumbs that fall from the Master's table. But when we pray, we are standing in the palace, on the glittering floor of the great King's own reception room. We stand where angels bow with veiled faces, where the cherubim and seraphim adore. Shall we come there with stunted requests, and narrow and contracted faith? He distributes gold! Do not bring before God stinted petitions and narrow desires. Remember: As high as the heavens are above the earth, so high are His ways above your ways and His thoughts above your thoughts. Ask for great things, for you are before a great throne of grace.

CHARLES H. SPURGEON

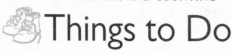

Things to Do

Helpful Hints for Buying Maternity Clothes

Before buying maternity clothing, check closets for loose-fitting exercise or casual-wear tops you already own that may be appropriate over maternity pants and skirts.

Most women wear the same size in maternity clothing as they do in regular clothing.

Clothes should fit loosely and hang from the shoulders for comfort.

Since you will be wearing maternity clothes only five or six months, it is sensible to choose wisely and borrow any that you can. When borrowing, keep a list to return clothes to proper owners. Or with permission, write the initials of the owners on the clothing tags using a laundry marking pen.

Don't purchase all of your maternity clothes in the beginning. Most women who have been pregnant agree that buying one new outfit during the seventh or eighth month gives a boost to morale.

A pregnant woman can look and feel fashionable with a few well-chosen dresses, some skirts, pants, and some pretty tops for dressy occasions. For everyday wear, elastic and Velcro can be used to adjust waistbands on regular jeans. Or buy a couple of pairs of maternity jeans or sweatpants and one or two easy-care tops.

A long dress, full and high-waisted, or one with a full skirt works well for most women. Full-cut jumpers are pretty too.

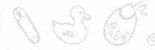

Bare shoulders in summer will show the part of you not enlarged by pregnancy and make you feel cool and pretty. Narrow skirts with maternity stretch in front or maternity leggings will help balance out your larger top.

Wraparound skirts are handy and pretty and adjust nicely at the waistline.

A long V-necked sweater works well for a top in winter. A man's big shirt will be comfortable for home wear.

If you can't find what you want in maternity shops, look on large-sized women's racks in department stores.

To keep a smart proud-to-be-pregnant look, buy or borrow classy necklaces, scarves, earrings, bracelets, and headbands to match maternity outfits.

You will probably need a support bra by the fourth month. The bust line may increase one or two sizes as maternity progresses.

Dress up in your finest wear and have Dad or a friend snap a full body photo three or four times during your pregnancy. In a few months or years, you won't believe you really looked like that.

TAKING

ACTION

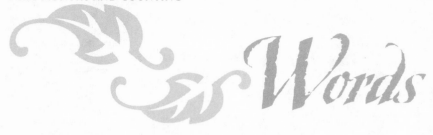

Words

Samuel was ministering before the Lord—a boy wearing a linen ephod. Each year his mother made him a little robe and took it to him. The boy Samuel grew up in the presence of the Lord.

1 SAMUEL 2:18-19, 21, NIV

David comforted Bathsheba, his wife, and slept with her. She became pregnant and gave birth to a son, and they named him Solomon. The Lord loved the child and sent word through Nathan the prophet that his name should be Jedidiah—"beloved of the Lord"—because the Lord loved him.

2 SAMUEL 12:24-25, NLT

Take a new grip with your tired hands and stand firm on your shaky legs. Mark out a straight path for your feet. . . become strong.

HEBREWS 12:12-13, NLT

My Presence will go with you, and I will give you rest.

EXODUS 33:14, NIV

to Live By

I command you—be strong and courageous! Do not be afraid or discouraged. For the Lord your God is with you wherever you go.

JOSHUA 1:9, NLT

Think upon me, my God, for good.

NEHEMIAH 5:19, KJV

In your strength I can crush an army; with my God I can scale any wall.

PSALM 18:29, NLT

The Lord himself watches over you! The Lord stands beside you as your protective shade. The Lord keeps watch over you as you come and go.

PSALM 121:5, 8, NLT

Great is the Lord, who enjoys helping his servant.

PSALM 35:27, NLT

How can we understand the road we travel? It is the Lord who directs our steps.

PROVERBS 20:24, NLT

[*He*] is able to do exceeding abundantly above all that we ask or think.

EPHESIANS 3:20, KJV

Is God's comfort too little for you? Is his gentle word not enough? What has captured your reason? What has weakened your vision?

JOB 15:11-12, NLT

What time I am afraid, I will trust in thee.

PSALM 56:3, KJV

The Lord is my shepherd; I have everything I need.

PSALM 23:1, NLT

The Lord is close to the brokenhearted. . . . The righteous face many troubles, but the Lord rescues them from each and every one.

PSALM 34:18-19, NLT

Day and night, I have only tears. . . . My heart is breaking. . . . Why am I discouraged? Why so sad? I will put my hope in God! I will praise him again—my Savior and my God!

PSALM 42:3-6, NLT

Through each day the Lord pours his unfailing love upon me, and through each night I sing his songs, praying to God who gives me life. I will put my hope in God! I will praise him again.

PSALM 42:8, 11, NLT

Your steadfast love, O Lord, [holds] me up. When the cares of my heart are many, your consolations cheer my soul.

PSALM 94:18-19, NRSV

God is our refuge and strength, a very present help in trouble. Therefore we will not fear, though the earth should change, though the mountains shake in the heart of the sea; though its waters roar and foam, though the mountains tremble with its tumult. There is a river whose streams make glad the city of God, the holy habitation of the Most High. God is in the midst of the city; it shall not be moved; God will help it when the morning dawns.

PSALM 46:1-5, NRSV

Do not be afraid, for I have ransomed you. I have called you by name; you are mine. When you go through deep waters and great trouble, I will be with you. When you go through rivers of difficulty, you will not drown!

ISAIAH 43:1-2, NLT

So don't worry about tomorrow, for tomorrow will bring its own worries. Today's trouble is enough for today.

MATTHEW 6:34, NLT

"Worth Repeating"

"A lot of people are willing to give mothers advice when what they really need is help."

"Today, I am too busy not to pray."

UNKNOWN

"The history of humanity is not the history of its wars, but the history of its households."

JOHN RUSKIN

"If evolution really works as some say, how come mothers have only two hands?"

ED DUSSAULT

"Next week, there can't be any crisis. My schedule is already full."

MOTHER OF TWINS

"In learning to walk with God, there is always the difficulty of getting into His stride, but once we have done so, the only characteristic that exhibits itself is the very life of God Himself. The individual person is merged into a personal oneness with God, and then God's stride and His power alone are exhibited. It is God's Spirit that changes the atmosphere of our way of looking at things, and then things begin to be possible which before were impossible."

OSWALD CHAMBERS

"I feel like a cow; I haven't gotten angry in weeks. I am
happy and contented. That satisfied smile must be
driving some of my friends crazy with envy, or at least
I hope it is. For the first time in my life, I have an
excuse for being plump. I am round and soft looking.
Yeah, no one expects me to be sylphlike."

ANGELA BARRON MCBRIDE

"Ye fearful saints, fresh courage take;
the clouds ye so much dread
Are big with mercy, and shall break
in blessings on your head."

WILLIAM COWPER, "GOD MOVES IN A MYSTERIOUS WAY"

"As a mother, my job is to take care of what is possible
and trust God with the impossible."

RUTH BELL GRAHAM

"Be strong!
We are not here to play, to dream, to drift;
We have hard work to do and loads to lift;
Shun not the struggle—face it; 'tis God's gift."

MALTBIE D. BABCOCK

THINGS TO KNOW

In the later months, you can actually see your belly move—a reminder that you are never alone. Somebody else is in there! Other people too can feel the action by placing hands on your expanding baby bulge. In the final four or five weeks, you will likely see the shape of your abdomen shift to the point of becoming lopsided and uneven as you are poked and prodded from within by tiny and precious elbows and knees. Such a phenomenon!

When I allowed family members to place hands on my belly to feel and see movement, they said: _____

_____

By the eighth month, unborn babies often react to external noises. Circumstances and sounds sometimes produce quick arm and leg movements clearly felt by Mom: "I was standing in the front yard talking to my neighbor. Her puppy ran barking toward the road followed by her three-year-old, and a car was coming. Frantic Leora shouted loudly at both to come back. She clapped and yelled again. Both times my baby inside jumped as if startled by all the racket.

During the last days of pregnancy, as the remaining time in the womb decreases, most babies will settle into the head-down (vertex) position getting ready to be born. This usually happens about two weeks prior to birth. The fit now becomes extremely snug, and freewheeling head-over-heels movement is nearly impossible, although some action can still be felt because Baby is still active within his tight quarters.

Did you know that the most frequently given name in the world is Mohammed?

Patience is difficult these last days.

There is a new life growing inside

that is nearly perfected.

A new human being will soon come forth.

The Lord has done glorious things!

Songs of victory will soon be sung in your camp.

Sit for a while by yourself in the sun. Feel its warmth flow over the two of you, then bask also in the sunshine of God's love for both you and your baby.

Thank God for simple things your mother or grandmother may not have enjoyed when caring for their babies: wipes, Kleenex, disposable diapers, dishwasher, automatic washer and dryer, running water. Others you can think of:

_____

_____

There is rich inner life there in your belly! Pause a moment to imagine your lower body opening for Baby to emerge with strong cries of life and joyful kicking. Your part is the pain of pushing, and you willingly help because you know the precious gift that will come from the struggle. Because it is true, repeat aloud, "The pain is a natural heritage. It is worth it all."

If I could give pregnancy a different name, it would be: _____

_____

Time with God

Prayer & Meditation

Lord, how can this be? A real person inside me!
A child that will have to come out!
This new life actually takes up space and is growing hour by hour,
with new cells, new blood, new muscle, new skin, hair and bone—all of
these marvelous increases coming out of nowhere to enhance my baby's size.
Sometimes this journey into motherhood seems so amazing,
so astounding, that it doesn't seem real—feels more like fiction—because
all of these incredible events are going on in a perfectly ordered way
in my deepest and most intimate private parts
where no one can see, not even me.
But then, when I planted my spring garden,
it didn't look any different for a while afterward either.
Lord, you were the faithful and skillful Master Gardener
who eventually brought all my seeds into fruition.
You are the skillful Master Creator of my baby too.

Almighty God, we give thee humble thanks for that thou has been graciously pleased to preserve, through the great pain and peril of childbirth, this woman, thy servant, who desireth now to offer her praises and thanksgiving unto thee.

BOOK OF COMMON PRAYER

Speak with faith about the birth of your baby: . . . I'm looking forward to the birth of the child within. I know God promises to be with me continually, and so I am not afraid. I know God will bless me with calmness and strength.

MARI HANES

Find a prayer partner, someone who will be praying for you and Baby in the next few weeks and months and who will promise to intercede for you during the hours of labor and delivery.

Write your own prayer for a healthy baby:

_____

_____

Write your own prayer for a speedy and safe delivery:

_____

_____

Things to Do

Many doctors recommend that pregnant women develop an attitude and pattern of resting often whenever they can because it increases the flow of blood nutrients and oxygen to the baby. This sensible habit can handily carry over after Baby is born so that Mom will lie down when she needs to, without guilt. Even ten minutes of napping does wonders once you get the hang of it. So go ahead and put your feet up!

Is your mom or aunt or best friend planning a baby shower? For laughs, have the invitation suggest that all guests show up looking pregnant. Each can stuff her clothes with pillows. You will feel tiny compared to some of your guests who will come looking like baby blimps because they love to clown around.

Give each guest a square of cloth ahead of time to appliqué or embroider with a personal message. The hostess or some other creative woman can assemble the squares into a crib quilt to be given as a gift for the mother-to-be. One woman asked guests to stitch up other matching items, a teddy bear, crib bumper, crib sheets, pillowcases, and wall hangings for the nursery.

If someone asks what type of baby shower you would like, suggest a coed event. Dad will enjoy it too.

For someone living far away, a videotaped long-distance shower can work even though the guest of honor cannot be there in person. The tape will surely be memorable enough to be played over and over. Fragile gifts can be mailed to the mother-to-be packed inside a box of diapers.

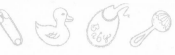

If guests are giving one large-sized shower gift, it will be cheaper to wrap it in a plastic or paper tablecloth printed with teddy bears or delicate flowers than to buy expensive wrapping paper. The tablecloth will come in handy later for picnics.

Shower game: Have each guest bring a baby picture to be hung on a bulletin board. Players get fifteen minutes to guess the identity of each baby. A prize goes to the guest who guesses the most pictures correctly.

More baby shower ideas: Here are wonderful ideas hostesses have worked out with their other moms-to-be to make baby showers festive and memorable.

The shower invitation can include a note to each woman asking that she attach an inexpensive baby toy to her gift. Mom removes them as she opens presents and takes them home in a pretty basket. One hostess floated a rubber ducky in the punch bowl and decorated the room with soft toys, bibs, rattles, baby bottles, nipples, and other small baby items. Of course, all decorations went home with the guest of honor.

The invitations can request that each woman bring along a self-addressed, stamped envelope with a blank sheet of paper inside to make it easy for the guest of honor when sending thank-you notes. Envelopes can be placed in a pretty bowl as guests arrive and used to draw names for a door prize.

A colorful balloon makes a unique shower invitation. Inflate it, then write the information on it using a Magic Marker. Deflate the balloon and stuff it inside an envelope with instructions to blow up the balloon for an important message.

THE
ARRIVAL

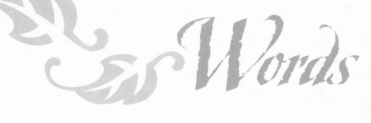

Words

Don't be impatient for the Lord to act! Travel steadily along his path.

PSALM 37:34, NLT

Bless the Lord, who is my rock. He gives me strength. . . . He is my loving ally . . . my deliverer.

PSALM 144:1-2, NLT

My soul, wait thou only upon God; for my expectation is from him.

PSALM 62:5, KJV

Before she goes into labor, she gives birth; before the pains come upon her, she delivers a son. Who has ever heard of such a thing? . . . Do I bring to the moment of birth and not give delivery?

ISAIAH 66:7-9, NIV

Can a mother forget the baby at her breast and have no compassion on the child she has borne?

ISAIAH 49:14, NIV

to Live By

Scripture praise prayer for my baby:

Praise God in his heavenly dwelling;
praise him in his mighty heaven!
Praise him for his mighty works;
praise his unequaled greatness!
Praise him with a blast of the trumpet;
praise him with the lyre and harp!
Praise him with the tambourine and dancing;
praise him with stringed instruments and flutes!
Praise him with a clash of cymbals; . . .
Let everything that lives sing praise to the Lord!
Praise the Lord!

PSALM 150, NLT

I will strengthen the weak.

EZEKIEL 34:16, NRSV

You will grieve, but your grief will suddenly turn to wonderful joy when you see me [Jesus] again. It will be like a woman experiencing the pains of labor. When her child is born, her anguish gives place to joy because she has brought a new person into the world.

JOHN 16:20-21, NLT

We know that all creation has been groaning as in the pains of childbirth right up to the present time. And even we Christians, although we have the Holy Spirit within us as a foretaste of future glory, also groan to be released from pain and suffering. O God . . . I trust in God . . . so why should I be afraid?

ROMANS 8:22-23; PSALM 56:4, NLT

Commit everything you do to the Lord. Trust him, and he will help you. Be still in the presence of the Lord, and wait patiently for him to act.

PSALM 37:5, 7, NLT

As pressure and stress bear down on me . . . you are near, O Lord.

PSALM 119:143, 151, NLT

Come unto me, all ye that labour and are heavy laden, and I will give you rest. Take my yoke upon you, and learn of me . . . and ye shall find rest unto your souls. For my yoke is easy, and my burden is light.

MATTHEW 11:28-30, KJV

I know the Lord is always with me. I will not be shaken, for he is right beside me. . . . My body rests in hope.

ACTS 2:25-26, NLT

I am focusing all my energies on this one thing: Forgetting the past and looking forward to what lies ahead. . . . Let us run with endurance the race that God has set before us. We do this by keeping our eyes on Jesus, on whom our faith depends from start to finish.

PHILIPPIANS 3:13, HEBREWS 12:1-2, NLT

"Worth Repeating"

"When Baby leaves the womb on 'birth' day, you become a mother; the basic mothering skills arrive about two minutes later."

"Birth is the sudden opening of a window, through which you look out upon a stupendous prospect. For what has happened? A miracle. You have exchanged nothing for the possibility of everything."

WILLIAM MacNEILE DIXON

"When a child is born into the world, God draws his hand out from near his own heart, and lends something of himself to the parent, and says, 'Keep it till I come.'"

HENRY WARD BEECHER

"Every mother is like Moses. She does not enter the promised land. She prepares a world she will not see."

POPE PAUL VI

"A woman loses a child even in having a child. All creation is separation. Birth is as solemn a parting as death."

G. K. CHESTERTON

"Ah, what an incomparable thrill. All that heaving, the amazing damp slippery wetness and hotness, the confused sight of dark gray ropes of cord, the blood, the baby's cry. The sheer pleasure of the feeling of a born baby on one's thighs is like nothing on earth."

MARGARET DRABBLE

"I had been in labor for thirty-six hours and was finally ready to deliver my daughter. I was holding my husband's hand while I pushed. But then he told me to stop—I was hurting his hand!"

A MOTHER'S LETTER TO *McCall's*

"Our life is drawn out to full measure precisely by having to accommodate ourselves to the needs of others to whom we are committed."

JAMES BURTCHAELL

"It still wasn't the kind of love we had expected, the kind celebrated through the centuries. It was the kind of love that made you feel as if your day began when they went to sleep, but which also made you tiptoe into the bedroom at least five times a night just to make sure they were still breathing."

ROBERTA ISRAELOFF

"Birth
One final push
and you burst forth
wet and waiting,
your farewell to womb
and your hello to world.

Love's labor done
I gaze
awed to silence.

Your exit and grand entrance
cry for drum rolls
and angel choirs.

Nine months you've
kicked and squirmed
seen through my womb darkly.

Now face to face
I murmur mother sounds
and touch your cheek and chin.

Love, which bubbled underground
   for forty weeks,
   bursts skyward in a geyser
   and melts heaven's gates.

In one eternal moment
I hear angel choirs
echo my alleluiah
to your maker
and mine."

CAROL VAN KLOMPENBURG, *Loving Your Preborn Baby*

THINGS TO KNOW

It has been estimated that baby expenses the first twelve months will be about seven thousand dollars for food, diapers, furniture, feeding equipment, bedding, clothes, and daycare. On average, moms and dads will change about seven thousand diapers in the two to three years before Baby begins to catch on to potty training (some children take much longer).

When buying furniture for Baby's room, don't forget a rocker. It will make Baby's midnight feedings and crying spells a lot easier for Mom or Dad.

University of Texas Medical Branch researchers in Galveston discovered that a rocking chair's motion relaxes abdominal muscles, easing the pain and discomfort associated with a standard cesarean.

Baby's ability to hear is fully developed at birth, unlike the ability to see, which most experts say takes longer. Baby has no doubt heard the soothing *beat, beat, beat* of Mom's heart for nine months. Some experts say that is the reason infants seem comforted by the rhythm of subdued sounds like the purr of a motor when riding in a car, the whir of a clothes dryer or fan, or the tick of a clock. It is interesting to observe how babies who are concentrating on feeding from bottle or breast will often stop sucking briefly when they hear a soft rhythmic noise nearby.

Ready, set . . . wait. If you are all prepared, but Baby is late, relax and remember that is not unusual. The average pregnancy lasts two hundred sixty-six days from conception to birth. About seventy-five percent of babies are born within seven days (before or after) the expected date of arrival.

There is no thinking of birth as something casual.

The experience reinforces our belief that there truly

is a God and that he has created all of us.

We cannot create babies on our own.

Birthing is the liberation of the child from the dark prison of the womb into the light. The one who is sealed is being discharged. But relief comes for the mother too, with release of the tremendously heavy burden from her belly and sweet, sweet reprieve from pain. It is over. The job is done! The blessed cord that binds is broken, and a better, stronger tie of love between Mother and Baby is created. . . . "You [God] have freed me from my bonds!" (Psalm 116:16, NLT).

I will praise God for bringing me and my baby this far: "It is good to give thanks to the Lord, to sing praises to the Most High. It is good to proclaim your unfailing love in the morning, your faithfulness in the evening. . . . You thrill me, Lord, with all you have done for me! I sing for joy because of what you have done. O Lord, what great miracles you do! And how deep are your thoughts" (Psalm 92:1-5, NLT).

Baby, are you as anxious to come forth from the crowded womb as I am to have it happen? Maybe we are both counting the days.

God wonderfully strengthens us in our hardships and trials.

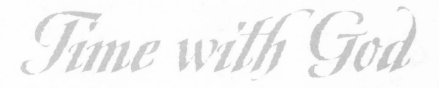

Time with God

Prayer & Meditation

God of grace and God of glory,

On Thy people pour Thy power;

Crown Thine ancient Church's story,

Bring her bud to glorious flower.

Grant us wisdom,

Grant us courage,

For the facing of this hour,

For the facing of this hour.

The One Year Book of Hymns, JUNE 18

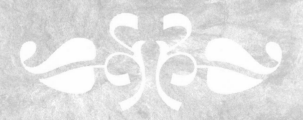

Lord, carrying this baby inside is one matter, but getting it out is quite another. Yet, I know it is you who prepared this lovely cocoon home for my baby, and it is you who handles the timing of my contractions, and it is you who will release her on just the right day, at just the right moment, in just the right way. I will claim your promise when labor begins: "I can do all things through him who strengthens me" (Philippians 4:13, NRSV).

Birthing a baby hurts. Pain is inevitable. Let the woman's distress be known, for her agony is real. Expelling the new life demands great strength. Her body must work hard. Crying out is the normal way to express the harshness of labor. Birthing is an experience like no other. One wise mother said, "Submit to the pain—yield to it—focus on the miracle it is accomplishing. You yourself are becoming a mother!" "In my distress I prayed to the Lord" (Psalm 118:5, NLT).

Right now, there are other women in labor, perhaps at the hospital or birthing center where you will be soon. Pray for their speedy and safe deliveries, healthy babies, quick recoveries, and strength to care for their infants when they go home. Ask God to increase their faith as they see what great things he does and how awesome he is in making babies and in creating the idea of families to raise them. Pray that the children will grow to love the Lord.

God, in a real sense, you too experienced pregnancy

when you birthed your beloved child, Israel, into being.

You are the great Deliverer too.

Did you not conceive the idea of the nation of Israel?

Did you not deliver your people from Egypt?

Did you not have patience for personally carrying them

through the forty-year wait in the wilderness?

Did you not deliver your beloved sons and daughters

(kicking and screaming and squirming!) into the Promised Land?

Did you not deliver Jonah from the whale?

Did you not deliver Daniel from the lions' den?

Did you not deliver your beloved Israel from captivity?

Did you not deliver Paul from the Judaizers and Peter from prison?

Did you not deliver me safely from my own mother's womb?

How often have you quietly sent your angels

to deliver me from trouble?

All so incredibly difficult!
I do not deliver this baby alone.
You know all about uneasy birthings.
You are the perfect partner in my labor.

Lord Jesus Christ, who labored on the cross for my benefit,
who gave second birth to many, bless me now as I too labor—
on this bed of childbirth. I know you understand.

The rush of waters when the amniotic sac breaks helps float
the cargo of the precious newborn safely into the world. Lord,
what marvelous planning! You are an awesome God!

A new life is born.

Things to Do

Make a list of all your successes, especially the things you do really well. Remind yourself that in a household with children, it is perfectly normal to sometimes be unable to see the bottom of the hamper for several days or to have children's toys scattered everywhere. That's just how it is. The perfect parent is a phantom, and trying to run your house like your mother did will only give you a headache.

Remind yourself how important you are to your family:
No job can compete with the responsibility of shaping and molding a new human being.

DR. JAMES DOBSON

Mothers are people too! Plan a break at home every once in a while, even if it's only a few hours. Hire a sitter or ask Dad to take charge of things while you just stay put in another part of the house doing whatever you choose:

reading a good novel, meditating on a favorite Scripture, polishing nails, trying out new makeup, finishing a quilt, or eating ice cream on the back porch with your feet up.

Swap a kid (or kids) with another parent, each taking the other's children for a few hours.

You will enjoy having company for dinner much more if you have a baby-sitter to take over Baby's care. The sitter can listen for crying and fussing while you relax with guests.

Ask Dad to bathe Baby today. He might enjoy it a lot. Sometimes men don't share in child-care tasks just because they never saw their own fathers doing them or because no one thinks to ask them.

Place a red-light, green-light sign on the front door so neighborhood youngsters will know when it is and when it is not OK to ring the doorbell. The green-light sign means it's OK. When the sign is turned to the red-light side, even little ones who can't read will recognize the signal.

Get up early to enjoy quiet morning hours by yourself before anyone else is awake (this may be the modern world's best-kept secret).

If you have other young children: Keep them busy while you rest. Give a child a deck of cards and ask her to sort by diamonds, spades, clubs, and hearts.

Assign an interesting drawer for the other child to explore in your jewelry case, dresser, desk, or lower cupboard. One mother keeps old spoons, dented pots and pans, oatmeal boxes, colorful plastic containers, or anything else she can allow her toddler to play with stored in the child's very own kitchen drawer.

Suggest the youngster use crayons to decorate lunch bags for older children or to draw designs on shopping bags for you or Grandma.

Add a little food coloring to soapy water in the kitchen or bathroom sink and allow the child to stand on a sturdy stool to play with it. Provide plastic dishes, a sponge to squeeze, or a soap bubble pipe.

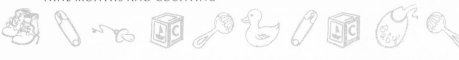

Young children often enjoy a toy made by inserting family snapshots into an old wallet. Toddlers will flip the pictures over and over and delight in pointing to favorite people.

Set your child in a huge cardboard box from a TV set or other large appliance with a box of crayons to decorate the inside walls. Ask him to create windows with curtains, wallpaper with designs, and a rug.

You can clip colorful plastic clothespins on the edge of a pan. Small children love to take them off, drop them in the pan, or replace a few on the edge.

Two- and three-year-olds love ripping old cloth. Ask your child to tear strips from a worn-out pillowcase or sheet so Dad can tie up tomato plants.

Some children can build all kinds of objects from toothpicks poked into gumdrops, corks, or marshmallows.

An indoor sandpile of cornmeal, oatmeal, or flour dumped out on newspapers on the floor can provide fun for a young child. Plastic cups and spoons, and small cars and trucks to tunnel through pretend roads and mountains will add interest.

A four-year-old will generally enjoy sorting buttons from Mom's button collection by size or color into compartments of an egg carton.

A percolator can make an ideal toy for a toddler who enjoys the fun of taking things apart and putting them back together.

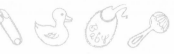

Fill a small canvas bag with knickknacks you find around the house to make a collection of terrific treasures to be enjoyed only at Mom's rest time.

A small youngster will have fun painting a concrete garage or basement floor with a paintbrush and a can of water.

Other things to do:
What fun for kids to announce a newborn brother or sister to friends and schoolmates in unique ways! One family announced Henry, their new son, by handing out Oh Henry! candy bars.

Ask older children to help design birth announcements before you go to the hospital or birthing center. Children's artwork is usually cherished by those close to the family. Or maybe you and the kids can bake and freeze cookies together with BOY frosted on some and GIRL on others (or do you

know Baby's sex ahead of time?). Youngsters will likely be excited to pass out the appropriate cookies at school when the time comes.

Let your child help announce Baby's arrival to church members by going with you into the sanctuary before the service begins and placing a perfect rosebud in a lovely vase on the altar table (be sure to arrange this ahead of time with the pastor). Children can help prop up a small nursery photo and a tiny typewritten card telling Baby's name, birth date, and weight. Remind them to tell youngsters in their Sunday school classes to come take a look.

A three- or four-year-old will love sharing with Dad the grown-up task of making calls to Grandma and Grandpa, aunts, uncles, and friends to announce, "Baby is here!"

Maybe older siblings would enjoy publishing their own family newspaper with headlines announcing, "It's a girl for the Johnstons!!" The time of Baby's birth, a description of Baby, Dad's thoughts, and others' reactions can all be included, as well as the expected date for Mom and the newborn to arrive home and who will drive them. Relatives and close friends will enjoy reading all about your family's big event.

One couple made a memorable occasion of finding out their baby's sex when they went together for her ultrasound carrying a beautiful antique box with a brass clasp. The physician was asked to write the baby's sex on a piece of beautiful parchment paper and to place it, unseen, inside the box and then to close the clasp tightly. The husband and wife carried the intriguing box to a favorite restaurant where they had courted, and talked a long time about the benefits of having a

daughter, then the benefits of a son. "Afterward, we agreed that whatever the sex, our child would be welcome, "she noted. It was a wonderful and unforgettable moment when the husband excitedly opened the box and shouted so everyone in the restaurant could hear, "It's a girl!"

Photo-smarts: Plan to have Dad or someone else take a picture of your newborn next to each gift and write thank-you notes on the back of the photos to save time. This gives everybody a glimpse of Baby too.

Bonus idea: Purchase an ink pad and stamp to date all photographs rather than spending time writing day and year on each by hand. Later, pictures can be sorted and filed or put in an album chronologically.

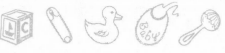

If Baby is overdue, rejoice in your preparedness and spend the time puttering, maybe clearing out a few drawers and rearranging shelves. Or catch up on reading, take long or short walks, rest on purpose, go out to lunch with a pal, or visit a nearby park or museum. Maybe you and Baby's father can take a one-day vacation at some nearby spot.

Why not design your own birth announcements to make them more memorable? Be sure to tuck one away in your pregnancy journal or baby book. You can address and stamp envelopes ahead.

AFTERWARDS

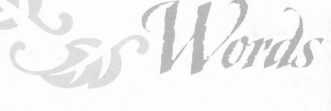

Give my [child] the wholehearted desire to obey all your commands, decrees, and principles.

1 CHRONICLES 29:19, NLT

We will not hide these truths from our children but will tell the next generation about the glorious deeds of the Lord. We will tell of his power and the mighty miracles he did. . . . He commanded our ancestors to teach them to their children, so the next generation might know them—even the children not yet born—that they in turn might teach their children. So each generation can set its hope anew on God.

PSALM 78:4-7, NLT

You [Lord] made me; you created me. Now give me the sense to follow your commands.

PSALM 119:73, NLT

Teach us to number our days aright, that we may gain a heart of wisdom.

PSALM 90:12, NIV

to Live By

Do not reject your mother's teaching; . . . a fair garland for your head, and pendants for your neck.

PROVERBS 1:8-9, NRSV

Bring them up in the discipline and instruction of the Lord.

EPHESIANS 6:4, NRSV

I pray that Christ will be more and more at home in your hearts [my children] as you trust in him. May your roots go down deep into the soil of God's marvelous love. And may you have the power to understand, as all God's people should, how wide, how long, how high, and how deep his love really is. May you experience the love of Christ, though it is so great you will never fully understand it. Then you will be filled with the fullness of life and power that comes from God.

EPHESIANS 3:17-19, NLT

How to behave so your children will too:

So put to death the sinful, earthly things lurking within you. Have nothing to do with sexual sin, impurity, lust, and shameful desires. Don't be greedy for the good things of this life, for that is idolatry. God's terrible anger will come upon those who do such things. But now is the time to get rid of anger, rage, malicious behavior, slander, and dirty language. Don't lie to each other, for you have stripped off your old evil nature and all its wicked deeds. In its place you have clothed yourselves with a brand-new nature that is continually being renewed as you learn more and more about Christ, who created this new nature within you. Since God chose you to be the holy people whom he loves, you must clothe yourselves with tenderhearted mercy, kindness, humility, gentleness, and patience. You must make allowance for each other's faults and forgive the person who offends you. Remember, the Lord forgave you, so you must forgive others. And the most important piece of clothing you must wear is love. Love is what binds us all together in perfect harmony.

COLOSSIANS 3:5-6, 8-10, 12-14, NLT

When I pray, you answer me.

PSALM 138:3, NLT

My voice shalt thou hear in the morning, O Lord; in the morning will I direct my prayer unto thee.

PSALM 5:3, KJV

Because he bends down and listens, I will pray as long as I have breath!

PSALM 116:2, NLT

A new command I give you: Love one another. . . . By this all men will know that you are my disciples, if you love one another.

JOHN 13:34-35, NIV

Love is patient; love is kind; love is not envious or boastful or arrogant or rude. It does not insist on its own way; it is not irritable or resentful; it does not rejoice in wrongdoing, but rejoices in the truth. It bears all things, believes all things, hopes all things, endures all things.

1 CORINTHIANS 13:4-7, NRSV

"Worth Repeating"

"The parent's life is the child's copybook."

"Every mother is a working mother."

"Sensing her husband's uneasiness about the time she spends with their fussy newborn, one busy mother uses Baby's monitor system to speak words of love to him if she knows he is somewhere her voice can be heard. Her caring words go a long way in easing the resentment new dads often feel."

"Babies are most affectionate when they have sticky hands."

"There is nothing cuter than a baby after all the company goes home."

"Families with babies and families without babies feel sorry for each other."

"The experienced parent is the one who has learned to sleep when the baby isn't looking."

"Your children are a gift to you. How you raise them is your gift to the world."

"Raising a child is like reading a very long mystery
story; you have to wait for a generation to see how it all
turns out."

"Who is best taught? He who first learned from his
mother."

THE TALMUD

"What the mother sings to the cradle goes all the way
down to the coffin."

HENRY WARD BEECHER

"Children are a poor man's wealth."

DANISH PROVERB

"A happy childhood is one of the best gifts that parents
have it in their power to bestow."

MARY CHOMONDELEY

"Children are like wet cement. Whatever falls on them
makes an impression."

UNKNOWN

"Children have never been good at listening to their
elders, but they have never failed to imitate them."

JAMES BALDWIN

"There never was a child so lovely but his mother was glad to get him to sleep."

RALPH WALDO EMERSON

"A baby is someone just the size of a hug."

ANONYMOUS

"Who is getting more pleasure from this rocking, the baby or me?"

NANCY THAYER

"While you can quarrel with a grown-up, how can you quarrel with a newborn baby who has stretched out his little arms for you to pick him up?"

MARIA VON TRAPP

"I love these little people; and it is not a slight thing, when they, who are so fresh from God, love us."

CHARLES DICKENS

"I tried to lead a child through play
To grow more Christlike every day
And I myself became that way."

MABEL NIEDERMEYER MCCAW

"Who was this immensely powerful person, screaming unintelligibly, sucking my breast until I was in a state of fatigue the likes of which I had never known? Who was he and by what authority had he claimed the right to my life?"

JANE LAZARRE

"In the sheltered simplicity of the first days after a baby is born, one sees again the magical closed circle, the miraculous sense of two people existing only for each other, the tranquil sky reflected on the face of the mother nursing her child."

ANNE MORROW LINDBERGH

"I often feel a spiritual communion with all the other mothers who are feeding their babies in the still of the night. Having a baby makes me feel a general closeness to humanity."

SIMONE BLOOM

THINGS TO KNOW

The *1988 Guinness Book of World Records* reveals that the unnamed wife of Russian peasant Feodor Vassilyev held the world record for producing the most surviving babies in a lifetime—sixty-seven! This woman labored over sixteen sets of twins, seven sets of triplets, and four sets of quadruplets between 1725 and 1765.

Experts say you will not spoil your new baby with a lot of holding. Newborns are not yet wise enough to try to control what you do. So plan to cuddle and hug whenever you can.

During the first six months, the baby has the rudiments of a love language available to him. There is the language of the embrace, the language of the eyes, the language of the smile, vocal communications of pleasure and distress. It is the essential vocabulary of love before he can speak.

SELMA FRAIBER

The Great American Baby Almanac touts that each baby is a genius— constantly observing, constantly practicing, constantly learning. There is no limit to infant curiosity, and a baby will often show equally dazzling speed of comprehension. Some of us are tempted to hasten the process along by more overt means than simple nurturing, but it is usually enough to let the infant proceed at personal pace; just the feat of learning to talk [later] makes every baby a Quiz Kid.

IRENA CHALMERS

There are two doctors who will assist

in the delivery of the child within.

One is the obstetrician you have chosen.

The other is the One whom Scripture names

the Great Physician.

MARI HANES

*P*erhaps we should sound forth trumpets and shout and sing loud hosannahs for the mother's labor. For when the squalling, wiggling, independent new body comes forth from the womb, a new human being has entered the world. One has become two—something unimaginably wonderful has taken place, something so extraordinary that it seems impossible. "Come, see the glorious works of the Lord!" (Psalm 46:8, NLT).

*T*ry to imagine the impact of birth—the amazing, immediate shifts in physiological functioning that enable the baby to maintain an independent life, the drastic change of environment with its barrage of new sensations. The baby's senses are assaulted by bright light and noise (including his own shrill voice); the feel of air on his skin, in his nostrils and lungs; the clasp of hands on his body; contact of instruments used to examine and ensure his welfare; the strange feel of clothing on his skin; even the sensation of his own weight on a solid surface; for his body has known only yielding surroundings.

The baby can't be expected to adjust suddenly to this new life. It takes time for the new functions now required of his body to become stabilized. Meanwhile, all these new activities—sucking for food, digesting it, emptying his bowels and bladder—tax his energy, and he'll spend a lot of time in sleep.

MAJA BERNATH, *Parents' Book for Your Baby's First Year*

Prayer & Meditation

Make [this child], O Lord, modest and humble, strong and constant,

to observe the discipline of Christ. Let [this child's] life and teaching

so reflect your commandments, that through [the child] many may come

to know you and love you. As your Son came not to be served but to serve,

may [this child] share in Christ's survice, and come to the unending glory

of him who, with you and the Holy Spirit, lives and reigns,

one God, forever and ever.

BOOK OF COMMON PRAYER

Lord, give my child the wholehearted desire to obey you throughout life, for that is the way to joy and fulfillment, whatever the circumstances. Help my child to realize that, because you love us, you outlined in your Word, the Bible, the best way to get the most out of life. Give my child a hunger for your word and a constant love for you.

Lord, I pray that my baby learns very early in life that there

is great reward for those who obey your commands.

If there must be trouble, let it be in my day

that my child may have peace.

THOMAS PAINE

Scripture prayer for my new baby:

Beloved, I wish above all things that thou mayest prosper

and be in health, even as thy soul prospereth.

3 JOHN 1:2, KJV

Are things coming at you from every direction? Since Baby's arrival, maybe you feel frazzled, pulled in a dozen different ways. It is important for new mothers to accept this fact as a very small and temporary inconvenience for so great a gift and not allow spiritual vim and vigor to lag with the physical. During the first weeks there usually isn't time for lengthy private talks with the Lord, but Mom can direct quick flash prayers while standing at the sink, bathing Baby, loading the dishwasher, pulling on mittens and boots for older youngsters, or waiting for a traffic light to change. "Pray at all times and on every occasion in the power of the Holy Spirit" (Ephesians 6:18, NLT).

Examples of flash prayers:

Lord, I draw now on your strength, your peace and calmness, to get this job done in the next few minutes.

Lord, I feel your presence. You are here. You are right beside me as I do these chores.

Lord, give me a spirit of acceptance and gratefulness for all the tasks before me today. There are a lot of women who would love to be able to do these things.

Lord, heal my baby's cold just as you healed the blind man in the

Bible and Jairus's daughter and so many others. You are able!
  I love you, Lord, because you hear my prayers and answer them.

Pray for a selfless attitude and patience as you care for your baby.
Recall how Jesus himself was a committed servant to others, and
pray for courage and a spirit of love as you go about daily tasks.

Write prayers for yourself and Baby as you begin this new phase of
life. Include your own flash prayers for strength and encouragement.

_____

_____

_____

_____

_____

_____

_____

_____

_____

_____

_____

_____

Things to Do

If you install a dimmer switch in Baby's room, a middle-of-the-night feeding and changing will be a lot more pleasant and peaceful. There is no need to hurt sensitive eyes with the glare of bright lights—getting Baby back to sleep will probably be quicker too.

In sticky summer weather, place a water bottle filled with cool water and wrapped in a soft cloth in the bend of your arm when you feed Baby. He can lie on the cool bottle while nursing or drinking from a bottle, and Mom will be more comfortable too.

If Baby gets fussy and needs nursing while you are shopping at the mall and you are uncomfortable nursing Baby in public, ask the clerk in a women's wear shop if you can use one of the private dressing rooms for a few minutes.

Every time Baby finishes nursing, pin a safety pin or stick a colored piece of tape on the front of the bra cup to help you remember which breast was emptied last.

A crying baby can be unnerving to everybody in the house. Once you have done everything possible to quiet your child, you may think he needs to be left to himself for a little while. Instead of just hovering nearby and listening anxiously, it is often better for Mom to find something to do like exercising downstairs, doing a bit of housework, or sitting on the porch with quiet music and a cup of tea. You can set a timer every ten minutes to check on things. Betcha Baby falls asleep! Some mothers record their babies' own crying sounds, then play them back during fussy periods to quiet their infants.

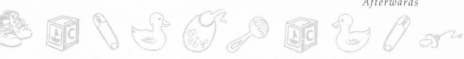

While you have Baby up for feeding in the middle of a cold night, place a hot water bottle in the crib. Of course, you will remove it before returning Baby to the crib. Baby will have a warm bed in which to go back to sleep.

If you experience leakage of breast milk, you can purchase nursing pads to insert in your bra, or you can make your own. Cut worn or faded flannel items into squares and fold them over several times; they will do a good job of absorbing excess moisture.

For information on breast feeding, support groups, one-on-one advice, and infant literature, write: La Leche League, 1400 Meacham Road, Schaumburg, IL 60173; or call 847-519-7730 or 1-800-LA LECHE; or visit their Web site at: www.lalecheleague.org

Before Baby arrives, clear your calendar of outside activities as much as you can, not only for the last days of pregnancy but especially for those weeks immediately after the expected birth date. You will need time to get to know all the wonders of your tiny new individual and to concentrate on the bewildering and wonderfully interesting new person you have produced. These will be your private and personal days to recover and get used to a completely new routine.

Wetting shoelaces for tiny infant shoes with a little water will help them stay tied.

Having trouble trimming an active baby's nails? Ask Dad or someone else to hold Baby while you do the cutting with blunt-ended nail scissors. If you have to do the job alone, you can fasten Baby securely in the car seat to keep wiggling to a minimum, or cut nails while he is sleeping.

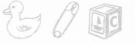

To save steps, keep basic baby clothing and other essential child-care items both upstairs and down. At the bottom of the stairs keep a lightweight basket with a handle. When you find things downstairs that belong upstairs, place them in the basket so everything can be carried up at one time.

During family times together, especially holidays when there may be several babies in one house, identify each one's bottles in the refrigerator with a strip of different colored tape, then pull the tape off just before feeding.

Bonus idea: Use bright nail polish to mark ounces on baby bottles so you can see the quantity more easily, especially during night feedings.

In the washing machine, pin tiny baby socks to a towel or other larger garment to avoid losing them.

Uncommon good sense: You will enjoy your baby more if you eliminate the goal of perfection in the day-to-day routine and replace it with the notion that people come before things. There is no need to prove anything to anyone. It is OK to leave dusting and cleaning undone and take a nap while Baby sleeps. If Baby's bottom is washed daily, a bath every other day may be all that is needed. The family will probably not even notice if meals are simpler or dessert is served only once or twice a week.

Some chiropractors recommend alternating arms each time you hold the baby to prevent the muscles of one side of your back from becoming strained.

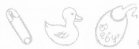

Bathing a slippery baby can be difficult. For the sake of Mom's back, it is sometimes easier for the first few weeks to use the kitchen sink (turn faucets away so Baby won't get bumped or burned). Place a towel in the bottom to keep her from slipping. Be sure to have all bath articles laid out before starting. It will be easier to hold Baby firmly if you wear a pair of soft white gloves; one glove can serve as a washcloth to clean Baby's tiny cracks and crevices too.

Set baby bottles in the refrigerator in an empty six-pack soft drink carton so they won't tip over.

Make faded receiving blankets do double duty by tearing them into small squares for cleaning up Baby's messy bottom.

Visitors will appreciate a waterproof lap pad when holding your new baby.

A plastic-coated shower rack or shoe bag hung on the wall near Baby's changing table can handily hold lotion, wipes, baby oil, and other small items within easy reach. Toddlers aren't so likely to grab them either. On a long car trip, the bag can be attached to one of the front headrests to store baby items.

Never, never leave a baby in the same room alone with a pet of any kind.

Many mothers say that during sieges of diaper rash, it helps to air Baby's bottom several times a day.

Pediatricians strongly recommend *against* heating baby bottles in the microwave. Microwave heating is uneven and often produces dangerous hot spots that can scald the mouth or throat. High microwave temperatures can also destroy essential nutrients. Heat bottles slowly in a pan of water.

Duct tape can mend a tab on disposable diapers.

Keep Baby's very own medical and health records in a small notebook in ink. Write in exact dates of all shots and illnesses. Later, this record will be very useful in filling out insurance and school forms. If you don't have time to record in the baby book immediately, tack up a chalkboard in Baby's room to scribble important information. Of course, everything can be easily erased after it is copied.

Repack Baby's diaper bag as soon as possible after arriving home, except for bottles and other perishables. Keeping it ready at all times saves a lot of hassle when you are getting ready to head out and allows you to go places on the spur of the moment.

Child-care experts recommend buying a diaper bag that is lightweight, with a comfortable feel to the shoulder, insulated, and easy to wash. It must fit in the stroller.

To enlarge holes in bottle nipples, poke in toothpicks, then boil the nipples about five minutes. Remove the toothpicks after the nipples cool. If the holes are too big, just boil the nipples without toothpicks to reduce the size.

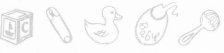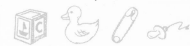

Stick up a sign that says "Day Sleeper: Do Not Disturb" near the front doorbell whenever Baby takes a nap. Baby will not be awakened and you will have uninterrupted time for yourself to sleep or do as you please. One mother leaves pencil and paper on a small table under a "Baby Sleeping" sign with instructions for visitors to leave name and phone number. She telephones to chat when time permits.

Lay Baby on a big sheet of newspaper or butcher paper, then trace a body pattern to take with you when shopping for clothes.

Things to Do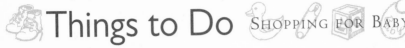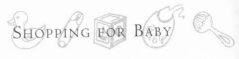

Shopping for Baby

Folks always seem to ask, "What do you need for Baby?" Sometimes Mom wishes she had a more practical answer on the tip of her tongue so real needs could be expressed instead of spur-of-the-moment ideas. Put these items on Baby's wish list, just in case you are asked:

• A stroller that converts to a carriage for use as Baby's daytime sleeping place (it can be wheeled everywhere you go in the house)
• A handheld cordless wet/dry vacuum to clean up spills or for use under the high chair later
• A cordless phone so you can talk while sitting in a favorite chair, feeding or soothing your newborn, or while walking the floor
• Lullabies on tape or in a music box
• Promise certificates for baby-sitting, house care, laundry, or cooking
• Gift certificates for diaper service, beauty care, or a night out for you and Baby's dad

• A gate to keep the family pet out of Baby's room
• A monitor for Baby's room

Check out garage sales and thrift shops for good used baby clothing. Babies outgrow clothes so rapidly that there are often nearly-new bargains. The unbelievably low prices will be especially appreciated if the clothes are to be used as back-up garments in daycare or when your child becomes soiled at night.

Stretch knit sheets are easiest to pull over a crib mattress. Small, washable waterproof pads can be placed in the middle of the mattress where Baby sleeps to save on laundering larger crib bedding.

Orphaned king-sized pillowcases will fit over the pad on the changing table. They are often on sale and pull off easily for washing.

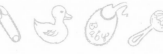

Buntings are easy to put on newborns and take off. However, it is impossible to fasten some car-seat buckles over garments that have no legs. Never buy a bunting without arms because you won't be able to securely grab your baby under the arms to pick her up.

Many mothers prefer plain stretch suits or pull-on plastic pants for Baby. Snaps rip off easily. Fancy pants trimmed with lace are often scratchy.

If you buy baby shirts, pants, sweaters, pajamas, play clothes, and other garments in the same color or in coordinating colors, you won't always be searching around in the drawers trying to match outfits.

Consider items that do double duty. Stores now sell a high chair that becomes a table chair, a portable crib/play-yard combination that folds into a bag for travel, and a stroller for use

while jogging. For day-to-day use, many mothers say front stroller wheels that swivel provide greater ease of handling.

Cribs with two movable sides cost more. One side that goes up and down is usually all that is needed, especially if the crib will be sitting against a wall.

A crib bumper will keep drafts away from Baby and protect her head. Plastic bumpers may not be as pretty, but they wipe clean easily (they do crack, however). Fabric covers get messy and often go out of shape when the bumpers are washed. For safety, the bumpers should tie or snap onto the crib in several places.

A cradle that rocks will probably need a bumper and should have a lock that holds it in place at night so Baby won't roll to one side and get stuck there.

Shopping List for Baby

CLOTHING

○ Diapers
○ Plastic pants
   (three or four pairs)
○ Sleepers
○ Socks, booties
○ Undershirts
   *(long or short sleeves
      depending on season)*
○ Bibs, terry cloth
○ Sweater, hat
○ Receiving blankets
○ Bunting or wrap

BABY'S ROOM

○ Crib, cradle, or bassinet
○ Mattress
○ Crib bumper
○ Crib sheets
○ Waterproof pads
○ Crib blankets
○ Dresser
○ Diaper pail, covered
○ Changing table
○ Rocking chair
   *(optional but
      recommended)*
○ Plastic baby-sized bathtub
○ Thermometer
○ Disposable wipes
○ Baby washcloths
○ Night-light
○ Laundry hamper
○ Baby monitor (optional)
○ Smoke alarm

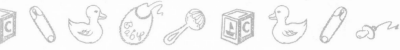

OTHER

○ Bottles, nipples

○ Bottle and nipple brushes

○ Nipple jar

○ Pacifiers

○ Nursing pads, nursing bras,
  breast pump
    (for nursing mothers)

○ Cotton balls, diaper rash
  ointment, skin lotion or
  baby oil

○ Infant car seat

○ Stroller

○ Baby comb/brush set

○ Insulated diaper and
  bottle bag

○ Fingernail clippers
  or scissors

Things to Do HEIRLOOMS AND TRADITIONS

For a treasured keepsake, write Baby a letter on the day he or she is born. Tell about the "birth" day's events, your feelings, and your hopes and dreams. Maybe Dad will do it too, or even siblings. Seal letter(s) to be given to your child years later, maybe on the 18th birthday, wedding day, or the day his or her own first baby is born.

You have time to plan ahead. Ask relatives the whereabouts of keepsake christening bonnets and dresses used previously by family members. Get the items cleaned and ready for use. Maybe Baby can wear a beautiful heirloom bonnet home from the hospital. (Later, embroider Baby's name and date inside the hem and make it a point to pass the things on to another family member when the time comes.)

If you have a family keepsake quilt gone ragged, snip out the beautiful places and stitch them together to make a keepsake coverlet for Baby's crib.

If someone is planning a shower for you, ask the hostess to have each guest draw a simple picture or write a note to Baby on white paper using fabric crayons. Part of the fun will be trying to draw or write the words backward since you will be ironing them onto white cloth to make a wonderful keepsake baby quilt.

Christmas pregnancy:
Invite everybody to join in decorating a teeny-weeny artificial Christmas tree that you have placed in the nursery. Let each child place a baby gift underneath the tree to be left until the expected newcomer is brought home. Living with the pretty tree and unopened gifts for a few weeks will increase the anticipation and excitement of bringing Baby home. Of course, older children get to open Baby's presents.

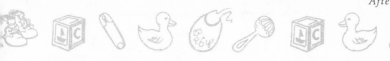

Let big siblings help bake up a batch of people-shaped gingerbread cookies, designing one for each family member. Baby gets an outsized super-cookie with extra frosting even though she is not yet born. Freeze and save the cookies for a "birth" day party with Mom when everybody visits her at the hospital after the big event. Guess who gets to eat Baby's cookie—no, it's not Baby!

Make a Baby Advent grab bag for the children to enjoy while waiting for the "birth" day. Tuck dozens of small wrapped gifts (candy, cookies, small games and books, dried fruit, dollar store goodies, etc.) into a pretty basket and allow youngsters to draw out one each day beginning about a month before Baby is due. Reserve especially enticing packages, maybe wrapped in gold foil, for Dad and the kids to open the first day after Baby arrives.

Make a big deal of wrapping a couple of Christmas toys for the baby-to-be and placing them under the tree. Help small children open them, then set them atop a high closet shelf for Baby. Help kids mark a date on a calendar when you think Baby will be able to play with them. Bet you can't count how many times they will ask, "Is Baby old enough for the Christmas toys yet?"

Make a Christmas bulletin board showing pictures of the infant Jesus. Cut letters from construction paper to tack up: "Our family is having a baby too." Have kids write letters or messages to Baby Jesus and to the baby-to-be for display.

Hang and fill a Christmas stocking for Baby during the holidays. In a few weeks, everybody will enjoy helping unwrap rattles and tiny toys to present to the little newcomer. Hang a Christmas tree ornament for Baby too.

JOURNAL

DATE _____ NUMBER OF WEEKS PREGNANT _____

_____
_____
_____
_____
_____
_____
_____
_____
_____
_____
_____
_____
_____
_____
_____
_____
_____

. . . how did I feel when I discovered I was pregnant

. . . how might my pregnancy and birthing differ from my
mother's

. . . what good memories do I have with my parents that I want
to re-create with my children

DATE _____ NUMBER OF WEEKS PREGNANT _____

_____

_____

_____

_____

_____

_____

_____

_____

_____

_____

_____

_____

_____

_____

_____

_____

_____

_____

_____

_____

_____

_____

_____

_____

_____

_____

DATE _____ NUMBER OF WEEKS PREGNANT _____

_____

_____

_____

_____

_____

_____

_____

_____

_____

_____

_____

_____

_____

_____

_____

_____

_____

_____

_____

_____

_____

_____

_____

_____

DATE _____ NUMBER OF WEEKS PREGNANT _____

_____

_____

_____

_____

_____

_____

_____

_____

_____

_____

_____

_____

_____

_____

_____

_____

_____

_____

_____

_____

_____

_____

_____

_____

DATE _____ NUMBER OF WEEKS PREGNANT _____

_____
_____
_____
_____
_____
_____
_____
_____
_____
_____
_____
_____
_____
_____
_____
_____

. . . how have my feelings changed from the time I discovered I was pregnant until now

. . . what thoughts do I have today that I did not have three months ago

. . . what kinds of problems have I encountered during pregnancy

. . . how have I witnessed God anew

DATE _____ NUMBER OF WEEKS PREGNANT _____

_____
_____
_____
_____
_____
_____
_____
_____
_____
_____
_____
_____
_____
_____
_____
_____
_____
_____
_____
_____
_____
_____
_____
_____
_____
_____

DATE _____ NUMBER OF WEEKS PREGNANT _____

DATE _____ NUMBER OF WEEKS PREGNANT _____

_____

_____

_____

_____

_____

_____

_____

_____

_____

_____

_____

_____

_____

_____

_____

_____

_____

_____

_____

_____

_____

_____

_____

_____

DATE _____ NUMBER OF WEEKS PREGNANT _____

_____
_____
_____
_____
_____
_____
_____
_____
_____
_____
_____
_____
_____
_____
_____
_____
_____
_____
_____
_____

. . . what personal issues am I working through during these months

. . . how does God help me during pregnancy

. . . what are some of the many blessings I am aware of today

DATE _____ NUMBER OF WEEKS PREGNANT _____

_____

_____

_____

_____

_____

_____

_____

_____

_____

_____

_____

_____

_____

_____

_____

_____

_____

_____

_____

_____

_____

_____

_____

_____

_____

_____

DATE _____ NUMBER OF WEEKS PREGNANT _____

DATE _____ NUMBER OF WEEKS PREGNANT _____

_____
_____
_____
_____
_____
_____
_____
_____
_____
_____
_____
_____
_____
_____
_____
_____
_____
_____
_____
_____
_____
_____
_____
_____
_____
_____

DATE _____ NUMBER OF WEEKS PREGNANT _____

_____

_____

_____

_____

_____

_____

_____

_____

_____

_____

_____

_____

_____

_____

_____

. . . what particular fears and concerns do I have today about pregnancy, birth, or motherhood

. . . how do I handle problems

. . . how can I see God's grace and mercy in my circumstances

. . . if I could give motherhood a different name, what would it be

DATE _____ NUMBER OF WEEKS PREGNANT _____

_____
_____
_____
_____
_____
_____
_____
_____
_____
_____
_____
_____
_____
_____
_____
_____
_____
_____
_____
_____
_____
_____
_____
_____
_____

DATE _____ NUMBER OF WEEKS PREGNANT _____

DATE _____ NUMBER OF WEEKS PREGNANT _____

_____
_____
_____
_____
_____
_____
_____
_____
_____
_____
_____
_____
_____
_____
_____
_____
_____
_____
_____
_____
_____
_____
_____
_____

DATE _____ NUMBER OF WEEKS PREGNANT _____

_____
_____
_____
_____
_____
_____
_____
_____
_____
_____
_____
_____
_____
_____
_____
_____
_____
_____
_____
_____

. . . what are my hopes for today/tomorrow/next week/next month

. . . which promises of God do I hold to the strongest these days

. . . what fun things have I done during pregnancy

DATE _____ NUMBER OF WEEKS PREGNANT _____

DATE _____ NUMBER OF WEEKS PREGNANT _____

DATE _____ NUMBER OF WEEKS PREGNANT _____

_____

_____

_____

_____

_____

_____

_____

_____

_____

_____

_____

_____

_____

_____

_____

_____

_____

_____

_____

_____

_____

_____

_____

_____

_____

DATE _____ NUMBER OF WEEKS PREGNANT _____

_____

_____

_____

_____

_____

_____

_____

_____

_____

_____

_____

_____

_____

_____

_____

_____

_____

_____

. . . how will I embrace motherhood—things I anticipate, things I will struggle with; hopes, fears

. . . what have I learned in the past that can help me with my pregnancy now

DATE _____ NUMBER OF WEEKS PREGNANT _____

_____

_____

_____

_____

_____

_____

_____

_____

_____

_____

_____

_____

_____

_____

_____

_____

_____

_____

_____

_____

_____

_____

_____

_____

DATE _____ NUMBER OF WEEKS PREGNANT _____

_____

_____

_____

_____

_____

_____

_____

_____

_____

_____

_____

_____

_____

_____

_____

_____

_____

_____

_____

_____

_____

_____

_____

_____

DATE _____ NUMBER OF WEEKS PREGNANT _____

_____

_____

_____

_____

_____

_____

_____

_____

_____

_____

_____

_____

_____

_____

_____

_____

_____

_____

_____

_____

_____

_____

_____

_____

_____

DATE _____ NUMBER OF WEEKS PREGNANT _____

_____

_____

_____

_____

_____

_____

_____

_____

_____

_____

_____

_____

_____

_____

_____

_____

_____

_____

_____

. . . who or what do I love

. . . who or what controls my life

. . . what am I afraid to give up for the sake of someone or something else

DATE _____ NUMBER OF WEEKS PREGNANT _____

_____

_____

_____

_____

_____

_____

_____

_____

_____

_____

_____

_____

_____

_____

_____

_____

_____

_____

_____

_____

_____

_____

_____

_____

_____

_____

DATE _____ NUMBER OF WEEKS PREGNANT _____

_____

_____

_____

_____

_____

_____

_____

_____

_____

_____

_____

_____

_____

_____

_____

_____

_____

_____

_____

_____

_____

_____

_____

_____

_____

_____

_____

DATE _____ NUMBER OF WEEKS PREGNANT _____

DATE _____ NUMBER OF WEEKS PREGNANT _____

_____

_____

_____

_____

_____

_____

_____

_____

_____

_____

_____

_____

_____

_____

_____

_____

_____

_____

. . . how will I train up this child in the way he or she should go

. . . how can I remember that parenting is for the kingdom of God and not just for me

. . . is there anything my child could do to keep me from loving him

DATE _____ NUMBER OF WEEKS PREGNANT _____

_____

_____

_____

_____

_____

_____

_____

_____

_____

_____

_____

_____

_____

_____

_____

_____

_____

_____

_____

_____

_____

_____

_____

_____

DATE _____ NUMBER OF WEEKS PREGNANT _____

DATE _____ NUMBER OF WEEKS PREGNANT _____

_____

_____

_____

_____

_____

_____

_____

_____

_____

_____

_____

_____

_____

_____

_____

_____

_____

_____

_____

_____

_____

_____

DATE _____ NUMBER OF WEEKS PREGNANT _____

_____

_____

_____

_____

_____

_____

_____

_____

_____

_____

_____

_____

_____

_____

_____

_____

_____

_____

_____

_____

. . . how will I set my child free to be all she can be

. . . what do I believe about discipline

. . . how will I show my child I love him

DATE _____ NUMBER OF WEEKS PREGNANT _____

_____
_____
_____
_____
_____
_____
_____
_____
_____
_____
_____
_____
_____
_____
_____
_____
_____
_____
_____
_____
_____
_____
_____
_____
_____

DATE _____ NUMBER OF WEEKS PREGNANT _____

_____

_____

_____

_____

_____

_____

_____

_____

_____

_____

_____

_____

_____

_____

_____

_____

_____

_____

_____

_____

_____

_____

_____

_____

_____

_____

_____

_____

DATE _____ NUMBER OF WEEKS PREGNANT _____

_____

_____

_____

_____

_____

_____

_____

_____

_____

_____

_____

_____

_____

_____

_____

_____

_____

_____

_____

_____

_____

_____

_____

DATE _____ NUMBER OF WEEKS PREGNANT _____

_____
_____
_____
_____
_____
_____
_____
_____
_____
_____
_____
_____
_____
_____
_____
_____
_____
_____

. . . what is the best thing about my home life right now is

. . . what is the most difficult thing about my home life right now is

. . . what were my thoughts and feelings when I first held Baby in my arms

. . . what fun things do I hope to do with this child

DATE _____ NUMBER OF WEEKS PREGNANT _____

DATE _____ NUMBER OF WEEKS PREGNANT _____

DATE _____ NUMBER OF WEEKS PREGNANT _____

_____
_____
_____
_____
_____
_____
_____
_____
_____
_____
_____
_____
_____
_____
_____
_____
_____
_____
_____
_____
_____
_____
_____
_____
_____
_____

About the Author

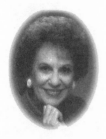

Alice Chapin has worked as a schoolteacher and has been on staff for Campus Crusade (military ministry) for twenty-three years doing seminars on family life and inspirational topics. Her previous books include the 365 Bible Promises series, *400 Creative Ways to Say I Love You*, *Great Christmas Ideas*, and *Hello Baby!* Alice and her husband live in Georgia and have four grown daughters.